Transgender Medicine

Editor

VIN TANGPRICHA

ENDOCRINOLOGY AND METABOLISM CLINICS OF NORTH AMERICA

www.endo.theclinics.com

Consulting Editor
ADRIANA G. IOACHIMESCU

June 2019 • Volume 48 • Number 2

ELSEVIER

1600 John F. Kennedy Boulevard • Suite 1800 • Philadelphia, Pennsylvania, 19103-2899

http://www.theclinics.com

ENDOCRINOLOGY AND METABOLISM CLINICS OF NORTH AMERICA Volume 48, Number 2
June 2019 ISSN 0889-8529, ISBN 13: 978-0-323-68119-3

Editor: Stacy Eastman
Developmental Editor: Meredith Madeira

Endocrinology and Metabolism Clinics of North America (ISSN 0889-8529) is published quarterly by Elsevier Inc., 360 Park Avenue South, New York, NY 10010-1710. Months of issue are March, June, September, and December. Periodicals postage paid at New York, NY and additional mailing offices. Subscription prices are USD 371.00 per year for US individuals, USD 761.00 per year for US institutions, USD 100.00 per year for US students and residents, USD 454.00 per year for Canadian individuals, USD 941.00 per year for Canadian institutions, USD 497.00 per year for international individuals, USD 941.00 per year for international institutions, and USD 245.00 per year for international and Canadian and foreign students/residents. To receive student/resident rate, orders must be accompanied by name of affiliated institution, date of term, and the signature of program/residency coordinator on institution letterhead. Orders will be billed at individual rate until proof of status is received. Foreign air speed delivery is included in all *Clinics* subscription prices. All prices are subject to change without notice. **POSTMASTER:** Send address changes to *Endocrinology and Metabolism Clinics of North America*, Elsevier Health Sciences Division, Subscription Customer Service, 3251 Riverport Lane, Maryland Heights, MO 63043. **Customer Service: Telephone: 1-800-654-2452** (U.S. and Canada); **1-314-447-8871** (outside U.S. and Canada). **Fax: 1-314-447-8029. E-mail: journalscustomerservice-usa@elsevier.com (for print support); journalsonlinesupport-usa@elsevier.com (for online support).**

Reprints. For copies of 100 or more, of articles in this publication, please contact the Commercial Rights Department, Elsevier Inc., 360 Park Avenue South, New York, NY 10010-1710; phone: +1-212-633-3874; fax: +1-212-633-3820; E-mail: reprints@elsevier.com.

Endocrinology and Metabolism Clinics of North America is covered in *MEDLINE/PubMed (Index Medicus)*, *EMBASE/Excerpta Medica, Current Contents/Clinical Medicine, Current Contents/Life Sciences, Science Citation Index, ISI/BIOMED, BIOSIS*, and *Chemical Abstracts*.

Printed in the United States of America.

Contributors

CONSULTING EDITOR

ADRIANA G. IOACHIMESCU, MD, PhD, FACE
Professor of Medicine (Endocrinology) and Neurosurgery, Emory University School of Medicine, Atlanta, Georgia, USA

EDITOR

VIN TANGPRICHA, MD, PhD
Professor, Department of Medicine, Division of Endocrinology, Metabolism and Lipids, Emory University School of Medicine, Atlanta, Georgia, USA; Atlanta VA Medical Center, Decatur, Georgia, USA

AUTHORS

JESSICA ABRAMOWITZ, MD
Assistant Professor, Division of Endocrinology and Metabolism, Department of Medicine, University of Texas Southwestern Medical Center, Dallas, Texas, USA

CASSIE G. ACKERLEY, MD
Clinical Fellow, Division of Infectious Diseases, Department of Medicine, Emory University School of Medicine, Atlanta, Georgia, USA; The Hope Clinic of the Emory Vaccine Center, Decatur, Georgia, USA

NOAH ADAMS, MSW
Consultant, Toronto, Canada

JENS U. BERLI, MD
Assistant Professor, Department of Surgery, Division of Plastic and Reconstructive Surgery, Oregon Health & Science University, Portland, Oregon, USA

ELI COLEMAN, PhD
University of Minnesota, Minneapolis, Minnesota, USA

TREVOR CORNELL, MD, MHSc
University of British Columbia, School of Population and Public Health, Vancouver, Canada

CAROLINE J. DAVIDGE-PITTS, MB, BCh
Assistant Professor, Division of Endocrinology, Diabetes, and Nutrition, Mayo Clinic, Rochester, Minnesota, USA

CHRISTEL J.M. DE BLOK, MD
Department of Internal Medicine, Center of Expertise on Gender Dysphoria, Amsterdam UMC, VU University Medical Center, Amsterdam, The Netherlands

JUSTINE DEFREYNE, MD
PhD Researcher, Department of Endocrinology, Ghent University Hospital, Ghent, Belgium

MARTIN DEN HEIJER, MD, PhD
Department of Internal Medicine, Center of Expertise on Gender Dysphoria, Amsterdam UMC, VU University Medical Center, Amsterdam, The Netherlands

KOEN M.A. DREIJERINK, MD, PhD
Department of Internal Medicine, Center of Expertise on Gender Dysphoria, Amsterdam UMC, VU University Medical Center, Amsterdam, The Netherlands

ELIZABETH S. DUDA, BA
Emory University School of Medicine, Atlanta, Georgia, USA

DANIEL D. DUGI III, MD, FACS
Associate Professor, Department of Urology, Oregon Health & Science University, Portland, Oregon, USA

MOLLY J. ELSON, BA
Emory University School of Medicine, Atlanta, Georgia, USA

LIN FRASER, EdD
Private Practice, San Francisco, California, USA

MICHAEL GOODMAN, MD, MPH
Department of Epidemiology, Emory University Rollins School of Public Health, Atlanta, Georgia, USA

OKSANA HAMIDI, DO
Assistant Professor, Division of Endocrinology and Metabolism, University of Texas Southwestern Medical Center, Dallas, Texas, USA

HEATHER S. HIPP, MD
Assistant Professor, Division of Reproductive Endocrinology and Infertility, Department of Gynecology and Obstetrics, Emory University School of Medicine, Atlanta, Georgia, USA

BENJAMIN KAHN, BA
Department of Dermatology, Emory University School of Medicine, Atlanta, Georgia, USA

COLLEEN F. KELLEY, MD, MPH
Associate Professor, Department of Medicine, Division of Infectious Diseases, Emory University School of Medicine, Atlanta, Georgia, USA; The Hope Clinic of the Emory Vaccine Center, Decatur, Georgia, USA; Department of Epidemiology, Emory University Rollins School of Public Health, Atlanta, Georgia, USA

GAIL KNUDSON, MD, MEd, FRCPC
Clinical Professor, Faculty of Medicine, University of British Columbia, Vancouver, Canada

SIRA KORPAISARN, MD
Section of Endocrinology, Diabetes, Nutrition and Weight Management, Boston Medical Center, Boston University School of Medicine, Boston, Massachusetts, USA

BAUDEWIJNTJE KREUKELS, PhD
Department of Medical Psychology, VU University Medical Center, Amsterdam, The Netherlands

BAO CHAU LY, BS
Department of Dermatology, Emory University School of Medicine, Atlanta, Georgia, USA

TESSALYN MORRISON, BA
Student, School of Medicine, Oregon Health & Science University, Portland, Oregon, USA

SCOTT MOSSER, MD, FACS
Director of the Gender Institute, Saint Francis Memorial Hospital, San Francisco, California, USA

JOZ MOTMANS, PhD
Ghent University Hospital, Ghent, Belgium

SASHA K. NARAYAN, BA
Student, School of Medicine, Oregon Health & Science University, Portland, Oregon, USA

MICHAEL F. NEBLETT II, MD
Resident Physician, Department of Gynecology and Obstetrics, Emory University, Emory University School of Medicine, Atlanta, Georgia, USA

TONIA POTEAT, PhD, MPH, PA-C
Assistant Professor of Social Medicine, Center for Health Equity Research, University of North Carolina School of Medicine, Chapel Hill, North Carolina, USA

JOSHUA D. SAFER, MD, FACP
Center for Transgender Medicine and Surgery, Mount Sinai Health System, Icahn School of Medicine at Mount Sinai, New York, New York, USA

JASON S. SCHNEIDER, MD
Associate Professor, Division of General Medicine and Geriatrics, Department of Medicine, Emory University School of Medicine, Atlanta, Georgia, USA

PAUL PARKER SCHWAB, BBA
Emory University School of Medicine, Atlanta, Georgia, USA

MARY O. STEVENSON, MD
Assistant Professor, Department of Medicine, Division of Endocrinology, Metabolism and Lipids, Emory University School of Medicine, Atlanta, Georgia, USA

GUY T'SJOEN, MD, PhD
Head, Department of Endocrinology, Center for Sexology and Gender, Ghent University Hospital, Ghent, Belgium

VIN TANGPRICHA, MD, PhD
Professor, Department of Medicine, Division of Endocrinology, Metabolism and Lipids, Emory University School of Medicine, Atlanta, Georgia, USA; Atlanta VA Medical Center, Decatur, Georgia, USA

OGUL ERSIN UNER, BA
Emory University School of Medicine, Atlanta, Georgia, USA

SHAWN WEN, MS
Emory University School of Medicine, Atlanta, Georgia, USA

BRITTANY L. WHITLOCK, BS
Emory University School of Medicine, Atlanta, Georgia, USA

HOWA YEUNG, MD
Department of Dermatology, Emory University School of Medicine, Atlanta, Georgia, USA

Contents

Accurate estimates of the number and proportion of transgender and
gender nonconforming people in a population are necessary for developing data-based policy and for planning and funding of health care delivery and research. The wide range of estimates reported in the literature is
attributable primarily to differences in definitions. Other sources of variability include diverse cultural and geographic settings and important
secular trends. The transgender and gender nonconforming population
is undergoing rapid changes in size and demographic characteristics.
More accurate and precise estimates will be available when population
censuses collect data on sex assigned at birth and gender identity.

This article reviews the current literature characterizing potential factors
associated with the etiologies of gender identity. The PubMed database
was searched for all literature that assessed key elements affecting development of gender identity. Current models attribute gender identity etiology
to endogenous biology along with prenatal androgen exposure. However,
no genetic loci or specific neuroanatomic regions have been consistently
identified as the single explanation for transgender identity. Although environment may play a role in gender expression, there are no data to suggest
an exogenous explanation for the development of gender identity.

For children and adolescents with gender dysphoria, an interdisciplinary
care team is essential for proper diagnosis and appropriate treatment.
For children who present with gender dysphoria, once puberty begins,
they can be treated with gonadotropin-releasing hormone analogs to
stop pubertal progression. This allows for further gender exploration, relief
of dysphoria, and better cosmetic outcomes by avoiding the physical
changes associated with puberty of the gender assigned at birth. After pubertal suppression, the individual may opt to proceed with puberty or start
treatment with gender-affirming hormones.

Transgender women often seek hormone therapy to attain feminine physical features congruent with their gender identity. The aim of feminizing hormone therapy (FHT) is to provide suppression of endogenous testosterone and to maintain estradiol levels within the normal female range. Overall, FHT is safe if provided under supervision of an experienced health care provider and has been shown to improve quality of life. Data on care of transgender women are scarce and high-quality evidence-based recommendations are lacking. This article aims to review the published literature on FHT and provide guidance to clinicians caring for transgender women.

Prescribing gender-affirming hormonal therapy in transgender men (TM) not only induces desirable physical effects but also benefits mental health. In TM, testosterone therapy is aimed at achieving cisgender male serum testosterone to induce virilization. Testosterone therapy is safe on the short term and middle term if adequate endocrinological follow-up is provided. Transgender medicine is not a strong part of the medical curriculum, although a large number of transgender persons will search for some kind of gender-affirming care. Because hormonal therapy has beneficial effects, all endocrinologists or hormone-prescribing physicians should be able to provide gender-affirming hormonal care.

The preventive health care needs of transgender persons are nearly identical to the rest of the population. Special consideration should be given, however, to the impact of gender-affirming hormone regimens and surgical care on preventive screenings. Providers should integrate a more comprehensive view of health when caring for transgender persons and address the impact of social determinants and other barriers to accessing affirming, inclusive health care. In individual interactions, providers must consider the unique impact that a gender identity and expression different from the assigned gender at birth affects patient-provider interactions, including the history, physical examination, and diagnostic testing.

Hormonal therapy and gender-affirming surgeries in transgender people have known deleterious impacts on future fertility using one's own gametes. This review focuses on fertility preservation, including the effects of medical hormone treatment on fertility, available and experimental options of fertility preservation in transgender adults, including sperm cryopreservation for transwomen and oocyte cryopreservation for transmen, and options for prepubertal transgender adolescents, including testicular and ovarian tissue cryopreservation. Transgender patients continue to face barriers and receive infrequent counseling regarding fertility preservation. Physicians should ideally counsel and discuss fertility preservation options before transgender patients undergo hormone therapy of gender-affirmation surgery.

Endocrinologists are at the front line for providing gender-affirming care for transgender patients by managing hormone regiments before and after surgery. This article provides the endocrinologist with an overview of the surgical options for transgender and nonbinary patients considering gender confirmation surgery, including feminizing and masculinizing facial, chest, and genital reconstruction. Discussions of the impact of hormones on surgery, and vice versa, as well as information on surgical decision making are provided to help inform patient education via the endocrinologist.

This review summarizes current studies, systematic reviews, and clinical practice guidelines regarding the screening, diagnosis, and treatment of osteoporosis in transgender persons. Gender-affirming hormone therapy has been shown to maintain or promote acquisition of bone density as measured by dual-energy x-ray absorptiometry. No differences in fracture rates have been seen in trans women or men in short, prospective trials. Trans children and adolescents on gonadotropin-releasing hormone may be at risk for decreasing bone density while not on sex steroid hormone replacement. Screening for osteoporosis should be based on clinical factors. Treatment for osteoporosis follows the same guidelines as cisgender populations.

Transgender persons receiving gender-affirming hormone therapy and procedures may face specific skin conditions. Skin diseases in transgender patients often are underdiagnosed and underrecognized despite their important impact on quality of life and mental health. This article discusses pathophysiology, diagnosis, and treatment of common skin diseases in the transgender populations. For transmasculine patients, conditions include acne vulgaris and male pattern hair loss. For transfeminine patients, conditions include hirsutism, pseudofolliculitis barbae, and melasma. Postprocedural keloids and other cutaneous complications are discussed. Unique aspects of skin health in transgender persons should be considered in the context of multidisciplinary gender-affirming care.

Gender-affirming hormonal treatment (HT) in transgender people is considered safe in general, but the question regarding (long-term) risk on sex hormone-related cancer remains. Because the risk on certain types of cancer differs between men and women, and some of these differences are attributed to exposure to sex hormones, the cancer risk may be altered in transgender people receiving HT. Although reliable epidemiologic data are sparse, the available data will be discussed in this article. Furthermore, recommendations for cancer screening and prevention will be discussed as well as whether to withdraw HT at time of a cancer diagnosis.

Worldwide, transgender populations are disproportionately affected by human immunodeficiency virus (HIV). Pervasive stigma and discrimination impact social and economic determinants of health, which perpetuate HIV disparities among transgender individuals. This article reviews the prevalence of HIV infection among transgender populations and presents psychosocial, behavioral, and individual level factors that contribute to HIV acquisition. The authors provide practical recommendations regarding a patient-centered approach to HIV/sexually transmitted infection risk assessment. The role of preexposure prophylaxis utilization in preventing the transmission of HIV is discussed as well as the current data on HIV treatment outcomes for transgender people living with HIV.

The field of trans health is fast growing, interdisciplinary, and global. The education needs of providers are also growing to keep apace of this expanding discipline. Scant education on trans health is available in undergraduate and resident curricula, or continuing medical education. In addition to the World Professional Association for Transgender Health's (WPATH) Standards of Care (SOC), Transgender Health Guidelines recently published by the Endocrine Society, WPATH has developed foundational and advanced educational programming in the areas of endocrinology and other specialties within interdisciplinary care. This article describes the history of transgender health care professional education and outlines the competencies related to this area.

ENDOCRINOLOGY AND METABOLISM CLINICS OF NORTH AMERICA

SERIES OF RELATED INTEREST

Medical Clinics
https://www.medical.theclinics.com

VISIT THE CLINICS ONLINE!
Access your subscription at:
www.theclinics.com

ENDOCRINOLOGY AND METABOLISM CLINICS OF NORTH AMERICA

FORTHCOMING ISSUES

September 2019
Pregnancy and Endocrine Disorders
Mark E. Molitch, Editor

December 2019
Endocrine Hypertension
Amir Hekmat Hamrahian, Editor

March 2020
Technology in Diabetes
Grazia Aleppo, Editor

RECENT ISSUES

March 2019
Thyroid Cancer
Michael Mingzhao Xing, Editor

December 2018
Hypoparathyroidism
Michael A. Levine, Editor

September 2018
Innovations in the Management of
Neuroendocrine Tumors
Ashley B. Grossman, Editor

SERIES OF RELATED INTEREST

Medical Clinics
https://www.medical.theclinics.com

VISIT THE CLINICS ONLINE!
Access your subscription at:
www.theclinics.com

Foreword

Transgender Medicine

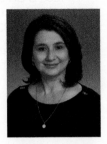

Adriana G. Ioachimescu, MD, PhD, FACE
Consulting Editor

The "Transgender Medicine" issue of the *Endocrinology and Metabolism Clinics of North America* is a collection of review articles that explore several important facets of this topic. The guest editor is Dr Vin Tangpricha, MD, PhD, Professor of Medicine at Emory University in Atlanta, Georgia, USA. Dr Tangpricha is an expert in the field and one of the authors of the Endocrine Society clinical practice guidelines regarding endocrine treatment of gender-dysphoric and gender-incongruent persons from 2017.

We dedicated the current issue to transgender medicine because of the significant increase in knowledge in this field in the past 10 years. Education of medical professionals plays an important role in improving health outcomes of transgender or gender nonconforming identity patients. Endocrinologists are at the forefront of medical care delivery for this population that poses unique health concerns. In the "Transgender Medicine" issue, epidemiology and biology of transgender or gender nonconforming identity are thoroughly explored. Current protocols of transfeminine and transmasculine hormone therapy are presented as well as information regarding gender-affirming surgeries. Several articles focus on bone health, fertility, mental health, cancer risks, and dermatologic conditions as they specifically apply to this population. From primary care physicians to endocrinologists, from surgeons to mental health specialists, and from trainees to researchers, this issue contains essential information on the topic of transgender medicine.

I hope you will find this issue of the *Endocrinology and Metabolism Clinics of North America* interesting and helpful in your practice. I thank Dr Tangpricha for guest-editing

Endocrinol Metab Clin N Am 48 (2019) xiii–xiv
https://doi.org/10.1016/j.ecl.2019.03.002
0889-8529/19/© 2019 Published by Elsevier Inc.

endo.theclinics.com

this important issue and the authors for their excellent contributions. In addition, I would like to acknowledge the Elsevier editorial staff for their support.

Adriana G. Ioachimescu, MD, PhD, FACE
Emory University School of Medicine
1365 B Clifton Road
Northeast, B6209
Atlanta, GA 30322, USA

E-mail address:
aioachi@emory.edu

Preface

Transgender Medicine: Best Practices and Clinical Care for the Future

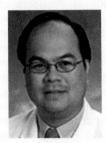

Vin Tangpricha, MD, PhD
Editor

There has been growing interest in the field of transgender medicine over the past 15 years. PubMed keyword text searches for "transgender" or the antiquated term "transsexual" yielded less than 50 entries prior to 2004. However, since 2005, there has been a steady increase in publications, which reached over 1000 publications per year in 2018. This growth and interest in the field have been largely due to increased awareness of the medical needs of transgender and gender nonconforming (TGGNC) people not only by the lay public but also by the medical community. Two important guidelines covering various aspects of the medical and mental health needs of TGGNC people by the Endocrine Society and the World Professional Association of Transgender Health (WPATH), published in 2009 and 2012 (revised again in 2017), respectively, have stimulated much of the recent interest in this field.[1–3]

While there remain many unanswered questions, we know that TGGNC people represent a much larger number of the population than previously believed. In this issue, Goodman and colleagues review the available evidence and conclude that up to 2.7% of the population have a gender identity that is transgender or gender nonconforming (please see Michael Goodman and colleagues' article, "Size and Distribution of Transgender and Gender Nonconforming Populations: A Narrative Review," in this issue). While the factors that lead to formation of a gender identity is not known, transgender identity is not a disease but rather a normal variation of human biology based on a variety of biologic factors, as reviewed in Sira Korpaisarn and Joshua D. Safer's article, "Etiology of Gender Identity", in this issue. TGGNC people have increased rates of mental health concerns, such as depression, and increased rates of suicide, which is likely due to mistreatment by society.[4] Gender-affirming therapies with hormones and/ or surgery appear to improve quality of life of TGGNC people.[4]

Endocrinol Metab Clin N Am 48 (2019) xv–xvii
https://doi.org/10.1016/j.ecl.2019.03.001
0889-8529/19/© 2019 Published by Elsevier Inc.

endo.theclinics.com

There are many published hormone regimens that can be used in children and adults, as reviewed in this issue (please see Jessica Abramowitz's article, "Hormone Therapy in Children and Adolescents," Oksana Hamidi and Caroline J. Davidge-Pitts's aricle, "Transfeminine Hormone Therapy," and Justine Defreyne and Guy T'Sjoen's article, "Transmasculine Hormone Therapy," in this issue). Furthermore, there are several protocols written on the delivery of primary care of TGGNC people as presented in the article by Brittany L. Whitlock and colleagues' article, "Primary Care in Transgender Persons," in this issue. However, many TGGNC people still lack access to health care providers who are adequately trained to provide culturally competent care (please see Lin Fraser and Gail Knudson's article, "Education Needs of Providers of Transgender Population," in this issue). Education programs like the comprehensive training course offered by WPATH, as an example, attempt to address the education gap among health care providers. Other special needs of the TGGNC population include skin conditions, fertility issues, bone health, cancer, and HIV risk (please see Michael F. Neblett II and Heather S. Hipp's article, "Fertility Considerations in Transgender Persons," Mary O. Stevenson and Vin Tangpricha's article, "Osteoporosis and Bone Health in Transgender Persons," Howa Yeung and colleagues' article, "Dermatologic Conditions in Transgender Populations," and Christel J.M. de Blok and colleagues's article, "Cancer Risk in Transgender People," in this issue). Finally, there is a need for more surgeons to be trained in the delivery of gender-affirming surgeries (please see Sasha K. Narayan and colleagues' article, "Gender Confirmation Surgery for the Endocrinologist," in this issue).

TGGNC people are individuals who have unique health care concerns that can be addressed following established medical guidelines. Increased training, understanding, and acceptance of this population will gradually improve health outcomes of this population. More research is needed in this field to optimize current hormonal and surgical regimens, improve mental health conditions and quality of life, and improve long-term health outcomes for TGGNC people. However, for now, physicians and health providers must use the best clinical practice guidelines available and provide care that is understanding and affirming when caring for TGGNC people.

Vin Tangpricha, MD, PhD
Division of Endocrinology, Metabolism and Lipids
Department of Medicine
Emory University School of Medicine
101 Woodruff Circle Northeast
WRMB 1301
Atlanta, GA 30322, USA

Atlanta VA Medical Center
1670 Clairmont Road Northeast
Decatur, GA 30300, USA

E-mail address:
vin.tangpricha@emory.edu

REFERENCES

1. Coleman E, Bockting W, Botzer M, et al. Standards of care for the health of transsexual, transgender, and gender-nonconforming people, version 7. Int J Transgend 2012;13(4):165–232.

2. Hembree WC, Cohen-Kettenis P, Delemarre-van de Waal HA, et al, Endocrine Society. Endocrine treatment of transsexual persons: an Endocrine Society clinical practice guideline. J Clin Endocrinol Metab 2009;94(9):3132–54.
3. Hembree WC, Cohen-Kettenis PT, Gooren L, et al. Endocrine treatment of gender-dysphoric/gender-incongruent persons: an Endocrine Society clinical practice guideline. J Clin Endocrinol Metab 2017;102(11):3869–903.
4. Nobili A, Glazebrook C, Arcelus J. Quality of life of treatment-seeking transgender adults: a systematic review and meta-analysis. Rev Endocr Metab Disord 2018; 19(3):199–220.

Size and Distribution of Transgender and Gender Nonconforming Populations
A Narrative Review

Michael Goodman, MD, MPH[a],*, Noah Adams, MSW[b],
Trevor Cornell, MD, MHSc[c], Baudewijntje Kreukels, PhD[d],
Joz Motmans, PhD[e], Eli Coleman, PhD[f]

KEYWORDS

• Transgender • Gender nonconforming • Epidemiology • Population

KEY POINTS

• Accurate estimates of the number and the proportion of transgender and gender nonconforming (TGNC) people in a population are necessary for developing data-based policy and for planning and funding of health care delivery and research.

• The literature addressing this topic spans five decades and presents data from 17 countries.

• On balance, the data indicate that people who self-identify as TGNC represent a sizable proportion of the general population with realistic estimates ranging from 0.1% to 2%, depending on the inclusion criteria and geographic location.

• Clinic-based studies seem to capture only a small subset of the TGNC population.

• Temporal trends show that TGNC population is undergoing rapid changes in terms of its size and in terms of its demographic characteristics.

INTRODUCTION

Accurate estimates of the number and the proportion of transgender and gender nonconforming (TGNC) people in a population are necessary for developing data-based recommendations and for planning and funding of health care delivery and

The authors have nothing to disclose.
[a] Department of Epidemiology, Emory University Rollins School of Public Health, 1518 Clifton Road, Northeast, CNR 3021, Atlanta, GA 30322, USA; [b] Consultant, Toronto, Canada; [c] University of British Columbia, School of Population and Public Health, 2206 East Mall, Vancouver, BC V6T 1Z3, Canada; [d] Department of Medical Psychology, VU University Medical Center, MF-H243, Van der Boechorststraat 7, 1007 MB Amsterdam, Netherlands; [e] Ghent University Hospital, Blandijnberg 2, 9000 Ghent, Belgium; [f] University of Minnesota, 180 West Bank Office Building, 1300 S Second Street, Minneapolis, MN 55454, USA
* Corresponding author.
E-mail address: mgoodm2@emory.edu

research.[1] In addition, accurate estimates of the TGNC population size allow developing social policy that protects against stigma and discrimination, inform effective transgender health care programs, and educate insurance companies on how to provide coverage for such care.[2]

In 2012, the Standards of Care for the Health of Transsexual, Transgender, and Gender Nonconforming People identified only a small number of articles attempting to estimate the size of the TGNC population, and characterized the state-of-the-science as at a "starting point" requiring further systematic study.[3] In recent years, several reviews sought to synthesize the available information regarding this issue[4–6]; however, the rapidly expanding literature warrants reevaluation of all available data.

In reviewing epidemiologic considerations related the size of TGNC population it is best to avoid the terms "incidence" and "prevalence" because these terms can lead to inappropriate "pathologizing" of TGNC people.[7,8] Moreover, the term "incidence" may not be applicable in this situation because it assumes that TGNC status has an easily identifiable time of onset, a prerequisite for calculating incidence estimates.[9] For all of these reasons we use the terms "number" and "proportion," which more precisely signify the absolute and the relative size of the TGNC population, respectively.

A total of 43 publications estimating the number and the proportion of TGNC people are available to date (**Fig. 1**). Of those 22 studies were conducted in Europe, 12 were based in the United States, two were from Japan, two from Taiwan, and two from New Zealand. Iran, Australia, and Singapore each contributed a single study. The years of publication ranged from 1968 to 2018.

The main findings from the available studies are summarized next. We discuss the evidence according to the definition of TGNC, which is divided into four main categories. The first category includes individuals who received or requested surgical or hormonal gender-affirmation therapy. The second category is limited to TGNC people who received transgender-related diagnoses, such as "transsexualism," "gender dysphoria," or "gender identity disorder." The third category defines the population of interest based on self-reported TGNC status. The fourth category is based on legal or administrative name or gender changes. The reported ranges for each category are

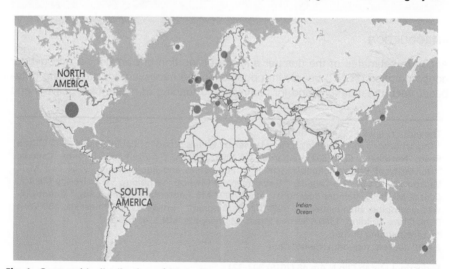

Fig. 1. Geographic distribution of 41 studies estimating the number and population proportion of TGNC individuals (*circle* corresponds to the number of studies from each country).

evaluated overall and separately for persons assigned male and female at birth (AMAB and AFAB, respectively).

In addition to summarizing reported ranges of TGNC numbers and proportions, we also discuss additional epidemiologic considerations that may contribute to better understanding of the characteristics and distribution of this population. Additional considerations include a need to distinguish between studies that were conducted in a clinical setting from those that were population-based, important differences in geographic distributions, and notable time trends.

PROPORTIONS OF INDIVIDUALS RECEIVING OR REFERRED FOR GENDER-AFFIRMATION THERAPY

Nine studies focused on individuals who received or requested gender-affirming treatment (**Table 1**). Of those, seven publications have estimated the proportions of TGNC people by considering only those who received or were referred for gender-affirming surgery.[10–16] The numerators for most of these estimates were based on clinical case series or surveys of practitioners providing transgender care, whereas the denominators were typically approximated from demographic data for a particular geographic area of interest. The estimated proportions of TGNC in general population in this category of studies ranged between 1 and 35 per 100,000 individuals. Note that these ranges cover a period of nearly 50 years, and come from studies conducted in a variety of settings and based on data of variable quality and completeness.

The corresponding data pertaining to the proportion of individuals who received hormone therapy are limited to two studies conducted in the Netherlands. In 1976, the Free Amsterdam University clinic established a gender team. Based on data collected through 1986, a total of 538 individuals began hormone therapy at that facility.[17] Of those, 399 were AMAB and 139 AFAB. Using the Dutch Bureau of Statistics data for denominator estimates, the proportion of TGNC in the Dutch population was calculated as 5.6 per 100,000 for AMAB and 1.9 per 100,000 for AFAB. In a subsequent study based at the same clinic, the analysis was extended through the end of 1990.[18] By that time, the clinic was providing hormone therapy to 713 transgender patients older than age 15 years, 507 AMAB and 206 AFAB. The total population of the Netherlands in 1990 was used to determine prevalence estimates of 8.4/100,000 AMAB and 3.3/100,000 AFAB.

PROPORTIONS OF INDIVIDUALS WHO MET THE CRITERIA FOR TRANSGENDER AND GENDER NONCONFORMING–RELATED DIAGNOSES

Of the 18 publications listed in **Table 2**, 13 studies calculated the proportions of TGNC people using diagnostic codes for "transsexualism," "gender dysphoria," or "gender identity disorder".[19–31] Methodologically, most studies that relied on TGNC diagnoses are similar to those that defined TGNC as having received gender-affirming therapy. Most used general demographic information to define the denominator and relied on clinical case series or survey of practitioners to determine the size of the TGNC population. The reported proportions of individuals with TGNC-specific diagnoses across populations in these studies ranged from 0.7 to 28 per 100,000. The corresponding estimates for AMAB and AFAB individuals ranged from 0.7 to 36 and from 0.7 to 19, respectively.

The numerators in the clinic- or physician interview-based studies are most likely underestimates because they primarily capture subjects who receive care at specialized facilities. Two studies (one in Taiwan and one in Iceland) addressed this limitation by using diagnostic interviews of the general population cohorts.[32,33] Both studies

Table 1
Number and population proportion of individuals who received or requested or requested to receive surgical or hormonal gender-affirmation therapy

Reference	Location; Time Period	Case Definition	Source of Numerator	Numerator			Source and Size of Denominator	Proportion (per 100,000)			Ratio AMAB/AFAB
				Total	AMAB	AFAB		Total	AMAB	AFAB	
Bakker et al,[18] 1993	Netherlands, 1976–1990	Receipt of HT	Free University of Amsterdam (AZVU) clinic records	713	507	206	Center of Statistics: 6,019,546 males and 6,252,566 females		8.4	3.3	2.5:1
Caldarera & Pfäfflin,[10] 2011	Italy, 1992–2008	GAS receipt	Surgical clinics	549	424	125	National Institute of Statistics 2009: total 59,619,290 (28,949,747 males and 30,669,543 females)	0.9	1.5	0.4	3.39:1
De Cuypere et al,[11] 2007	Belgium, 1985–2003	GAS receipt	Questionnaires sent to "gender teams" and plastic surgeons	412	292	120	January 2003 population: 3,758,969 males and 4,048,095 females		7.7	3.0	2.43:1
Dhejne et al,[15] 2014	Sweden, 1960–2010	Request (receipt) of GAS	National Board of Health and Welfare Statistics	767 (681)	478 (429)	289 (252)	December 2010 population: 3,704,685 males and 3,791,791 females	10.2 (9.1)	12.9 (11.6)	7.5 (6.6)	1.7:1
Eklund et al,[17] 1988	Netherlands, 1976–1986	Receipt of HT	Free University of Amsterdam (AZVU) clinic records	538	399	159	Dutch census data: 7,125,000 males and 8,368,421 females[a]		1980: 2.2 1983: 3.8 1986: 5.6	1980: 0.5 1983: 1.0 1986: 1.9	3:1
Esteva de Antonio et al,[16] 2012	Spain, 1999–2011	Request for GAS	Questionnaires sent to gender identity units	3303			Spanish population 15–64 years old, 33,030,000[a]	10.0			1.9:1

Pauly,[14] 1968	United States, dates not specified	Request for GAS	Author's communication with specialized centers		2000	500	200,000 total US population used for both AMAB and AFAB calculations		1.0	0.25	4:1
Tsoi,[12] 1988	Singapore, until 1986	Request for GAS	Documented diagnosis of transsexualism as part of pre-GCS evaluation	458	343	115	Population June 1986: 979,300 males and 954,900 females		35.0	12.0	3:1
Vujovic et al,[13] 2009	Serbia, 1987–2006	Receipt of GAS	Informed written consent to undergo treatment	147	71	76	7,500,000 (World Bank data)	1.96	1.89	2.0	1:1

Abbreviations: GAS, gender-affirming surgery; HT, hormone therapy.
[a] Denominator calculated from the numerator and the reported proportion.

Table 2
Number and population proportion of individuals who received a transgender-specific diagnosis

Reference	Location; Time Period	Case Definition	Source of Numerator	Numerator			Source and Size of Denominator	Proportion (per 100,000)			Ratio AMAB/ AFAB
				Total	AMAB	AFAB		Total	AMAB	AFAB	
Ahmadzad-Asl et al,[24] 2010	Iran, 2002–2009	GID diagnosis DSM-IV-TR	Tehran Psychiatric Institute	281	138	143	Center of Statistics of Iran, population aged 15–44: 39,526,948	0.7	0.69	0.74	0.96:1
Baba et al,[23] 2011	Hokkaido, Japan, December 2003–January 2010	GID diagnosis ICD-10 and DSM-IV	Sapporo Medical University Hospital	342	104	238	Native Japanese Hokkaido residents: 5,500,000		3.97	8.2	1:2
Becerra-Fernández et al,[29] 2017	Autonomous Region of Madrid (Spain), 2007–2015	ICD-10 and/or gender identity disorder based on the DSM-IV-TR	Patients referred to the GIU at the Hospital Universitario Ramon y Cajal (Madrid)	1171	803	368	Official population in the autonomous region of Madrid >15 year old in 2015: 5,310,409 (2,516,147 males and 2,794,262 females)	22.1	31.2	12.9	2.2:1
Blosnich et al,[34] 2013	VA system, United States, 2002–2011	GID diagnosis ICD-9 codes 302.85 (GID) or 302.6 (GID NOS)	Confirmed GID diagnosis in VHA, FY 2000–2011	2002: 569 2011: 1329			Total VHA patients: 4,544,353 (2002), 5,795,165 (2011)	2002: 12.5 2011: 22.9			
Esteva et al,[20] 2006	Andalucia, Spain, 1999–2004	GID diagnosis	Regional gender identity disorder unit		243	148	Regional Population: 2,359,223 males and 2,276,923 females[a]		10.3	6.5	1.64:1
Gómez Gil et al,[21] 2006	Catalonia, Spain, 1996–2004	ICD-10 F64.0 (transsexualism)	Psychiatric and Psychology Institute at the Barcelona Hospital, 1996–2004	Catalonia: Barcelona:	Catalonia: 113 Barcelona: 100	Catalonia: 48 Barcelona: 45	Catalonia: 2,376,538 males 2,308,611 females Barcelona: 1,996,708 males 1,776,269 females	Catalonia: Barcelona:	Catalonia: 4.8 Barcelona: 5.5	Catalonia: 2.1 Barcelona: 2.5	2.6:1
Hoenig & Kenna,[19] 1974	England and Wales, 1958–1968	GID	Royal Infirmary Manchester at the University Department of Psychiatry	66	49	17	Manchester population June 30, 1970: 3,498,700 (1,652,000 males 1,846,700 females)	1.9	2.9	0.9	3.25:1

Study	Location, Dates	Diagnosis	Sampling Method / Source	N	Subset	Population				Ratio
Hwu et al,[32] 1989	Taiwan, 1982–1986	Diagnostic Interview Survey	Multistage random sampling method	Taipei: 3 Small towns: 6 Rural villages: 3		Taipei: 5000 Small towns: 3000 Rural villages: 3000	Taipei: 60 Small towns: 200 Rural villages: 30	Taipei: 40 Small towns: 0 Rural villages: 0	Taipei: 80 Small towns: 420 Rural villages: 70	Taipei: 1:2
Judge et al,[25] 2014	Ireland, 2005–2014	GID, DSM-IV/V	GD clinic referrals 2005–2014	218		2011 census reports: total 3,205,882[a]	6.8	9.88	3.6	2.7:1
Kauth et al,[35] 2014	VA system, US, 2006–2013	GID diagnosis ICD-9 codes 302.85, 302.6, 302.5	Confirmed GID diagnosis VHA, FY 2006–2013	2567		VHA enrollees: 7,809,269		32.9		
O'Gorman,[31] 1982	Northern Ireland, dates not specified	GID	Clinic based, >14 y	28	21	Northern Ireland population: 1,500,000	1.9			3:1
Okabe et al,[22] 2008	Japan, April 1997–October 2005	GID, DSM-IV	GID Clinic- Okayama University Hospital	579	349	Inhabitants of Western Japan, estimated at 40,000,000		0.9		1.5:1
Quinn et al,[36] 2017	Kaiser Permanente, United States, 2006–2014	Transgender-specific diagnoses and free-text keywords	Electronic medical records at Kaiser Permanente sites in Georgia, NoCal, and SoCal			All members enrolled in a given year	2006 GA: 3.5 SoCal: 5.5 NoCal: 17 2014 GA: 38 SoCal: 44 NoCal: 75			2006: 1.7:1 2014: 1.7:1
Ross et al,[27] 1981	Australia, 1976–1978	Transsexual	Questionnaires to registered psychiatrists	243	209	Australia's population on June 31, 1978: 10,616,188[a]	2.4	4.2	0.7	6.1:1
Stefansson et al,[33] 1991	Iceland, 1931–1986	"Transsexual" diagnosis	Diagnostic interview schedule	1	34	862 persons representing half of the 1931 birth cohort in Iceland (441 males, 421 females)	100			

(continued on next page)

Table 2
(continued)

Reference	Location; Time Period	Case Definition	Source of Numerator	Numerator			Source and Size of Denominator	Proportion (per 100,000)			Ratio AMAB/AFAB
				Total	AMAB	AFAB		Total	AMAB	AFAB	
Wålinder,[26] 1968	Sweden, as of 1965	GID	Survey of psychiatrists	110			Not stated, estimate: 6,272,886[a]	1.9	2.7	1.0	2.5:1
Wiepjes et al,[30] 2018	Amsterdam, 1972–2015	ICD-9 and ICD -10 codes	Medical files of all people who attended the gender identity clinic	6793	4432	2361	Total population of people at least 16 years old in the Netherlands in 2015: 13,870,426	27.7	36.4	19.3	1.9:1
Wilson et al,[28] 1999	Scotland, 1998	GD	Questionnaires to general medical practices	273	218	55	Registered patients >15 y of age: 3,336,261 (1,622,090 males 1,714,171 females)	8.2	13.4	3.2	4:1

Abbreviations: DSM, diagnostic and statistical manual of mental disorders; GD, gender dysphoria; GID, gender identity disorder; ICD, international classification of diseases; NoCal, Northern California; SoCal, Southern California; VHA, veterans health administration.

[a] Denominator calculated from the numerator and the reported proportion.

administered site-specific versions of the Diagnostic Interview Schedule by the US National Institute of Mental Health. Although these studies were conducted several decades ago and may no longer be applicable, both reported proportions (range, 30–100 per 100,000) that exceeded those obtained from clinics or from surveys of health care providers. Note, however, that the estimates in both studies were statistically imprecise because they were based on small sample sizes and identified few TGNC people.

Several studies estimated proportions of TGNC people among individuals enrolled in health care systems. Blosnich and colleagues[34] used Veterans Health Administration electronic medical records from 2000 through 2011. The numerator for the study included individuals that had received an International Classification of Diseases-9th edition diagnostic code of either 302.85 (gender identity disorder) or 302.6 (gender identity disorder not otherwise specified). Using the Veterans Health Administration data and electronic record database to define the denominator, the authors reported prevalence estimates for different years starting in 2002. The 2002 estimate was 12.5 per 100,000 and the proportion reported in 2011 was 22.9 per 100,000. In a more recent similarly designed VA-based study the numerator was expanded to include International Classification of Diseases-9th edition code 302.5 (transsexualism). The proportion of TGNC veterans in 2013 was 32.9 per 100,000.[35]

Another health systems–based study evaluated electronic medical records data at Kaiser Permanente sites in Georgia, Northern California, and Southern California.[36] The numerator was ascertained using step-wise methodology, which involved computerized searches of diagnostic codes supplemented by a review of free text to identify TGNC individuals. The proportions of TGNC Kaiser Permanente enrollees increased over time at each of the three participating sites. In 2006, the estimates per 100,000 enrollees were 3.5, 5.5, and 17 in Georgia, Southern California, and Northern California, respectively; however, by 2014, the corresponding estimates increased to 38, 44, and 75.

PROPORTIONS OF ADULTS WITH SELF-REPORTED TRANSGENDER AND GENDER NONCONFORMING IDENTITY

Nine studies listed in **Table 3** used survey-based data to estimate the proportion of adults (persons older than age 18 years) who self-identified as TGNC.[37–45] The use of self-report greatly increased the likelihood that an individual would meet the criteria for inclusion in the numerator. The resulting proportions were also orders of magnitude higher and thus could be expressed as percentages.

In the United States, several studies took advantage of the Behavioral Risk Factor Surveillance Study (BRFSS), an annual telephone survey conducted in all 50 states and US territories.[37–40] One of the earliest BRFSS-based studies analyzed data collected between 2007 and 2009 in the State of Massachusetts.[37] The survey was administered to 28,662 adults, and contained the following module: "Some people describe themselves as transgender when they experience a different gender identity from their sex at birth. For example, a person born into a male body, but who feels female or lives as a woman. Do you consider yourself to be transgender?" A total of 131 participants responded "yes" to that question, corresponding to a proportion of 0.5%.

In 2014, the same BRFSS question was adopted by 19 states and the territory of Guam. Across all participating sites, TGNC individuals made up 0.53%.[38] An additional analysis of the same data estimated the proportion of TGNC population for the entire US by extrapolating data from the 20 participating sites.[39] The missing information for states and territories that did not inquire about TGNC status was imputed

Table 3
Number and population proportion of adults who self-reported transgender identity and gender nonconformity

Reference	Location; Time Period	Case Definition	Source of Numerator	Numerator			Size of Denominator	Proportion (per 100,000)			Ratio AMAB/ AMAB
				Total	AMAB	AFAB		Total	AMAB	AFAB	
Ahs et al,[44] 2018	Stockholm County, Sweden, 2014	Desire to undergo treatment	Stockholm Public Health Cohort study questionnaire	121	60	61	50,157; 21,586 males and 28,571 females	500	600	400	1:1
		Feeling as person of different sex		770	309	461		2300	2100	2500	1:1.49
		Desire to be treated as person of different sex		779	218	561		2800	2000	3500	1:2.57
Conron et al,[37] 2012	Massachusetts, 2007–2009	Self-identity as transgender	Massachusetts BRFSS 2007–2009	131			28,176	500			
Crissman et al,[38] 2017	United States, 2014	Self-identity as transgender	Annual cross-sectional telephone survey in all US states and 3 territories	TGNC: 807 Trans: 691	Trans: 363	Trans: 212	151,456 (62,086 cis-males, 886,679 cis-females)	TGNC 530 Trans: 456	581	238	2.4:1
Flores et al,[39] 2016	United States, 2014	Self-identity as transgender	BRFSS, in all US states and 3 US territories	1,400,000			233,333,333[a]	600			

Study	Location, dates	Definition	Survey			Sample				
Gates,[40] 2011	California, 2003–2009	Self-identity as transgender	2009 California Health Interview Survey, 2003 CA LGBT Tobacco Survey	49		47,614 survey participants in the California Health Interview Survey	100	600	200	3:1
Kuyper & Wijsen,[42] 2014	Netherlands, 2013	Incongruent gender identity	Sexual Health Survey	48	16	8064				
Lai et al,[45] 2010	Taiwan, University, 2003–2004	Self-reported gender dysphoria	Adult Self-Report Inventory-4, DSM-IV referenced rating	49	176	5010 (2585 males, 2425 females) first-year college students	4500	1900	7300	1:3
Reisner et al,[41] 2014	United States, 2010	Self-identity as transgender	Growing Up Today Study	10	16	7831 (2605 males, and 5226 females)	330	380	310	
Van Caenegem et al,[43] 2015	Flanders, Belgium, 2011–2012	Incongruent gender identity	Sexual Health Survey	7	6	1799	722	783	662	1.2:1

Abbreviations: BRFSS, behavioral risk factor surveillance survey; DSM, diagnostic and statistical manual of mental disorders.

[a] Denominator calculated from the numerator and the reported proportion.

using multilevel statistical models. Based on these calculations, the estimated number of TGNC adults residing in the United States in 2014 was approximately 1.4 million, which constitutes 0.6% of the total population (or 600 per 100,000). The state-specific estimates ranged from 0.3% to 0.8% in North Dakota and Hawaii, respectively.

Using the Growing Up Today prospective cohort study of US young adults, a 2010 survey implemented a two-step approach by inquiring about sex assigned at birth, and asking about the participants' self-described gender identity.[41] The response options were "female," "male," "transgender," and "do not identify as female, male or transgender." Of the 7831 survey respondents, 26 (0.33%) identified as having a gender identity that differed from the assigned (natal) sex. Of those, seven (0.09%) were cross-sex identified; five (0.06%) self-described as transgender; and 14 (0.18%) did not identify as female, male, or transgender. These data indicate that when assessing proportion of TGNC people it is important to include nonbinary measures especially among younger adults.

Kuyper and Wijsen[42] estimated the proportion of TGNC people among adolescent and adult residents of the Netherlands using Internet-based data collection. The study sample included 8064 participants who were asked questions regarding gender identity and gender dysphoric feelings (defined as ambivalent or incongruent gender identity, dislike of body characteristics, or wish to obtain treatment). The analysis of the data yielded proportions of 0.6% for AMAB and 0.2% among AFAB; however, the response rate was low (20%).

A similar study estimated proportion of TGNC people among residents of the Flanders region in Belgium.[43] Eligible participants were randomly selected from the Belgian National Register and 1799 (48%) completed the survey. Information pertaining to gender identity and gender expression was collected via a computer-assisted personal interview. Using a five-point Likert scale, the participants were asked to score the following statements: "I feel like a woman," and "I feel like a man." A person was considered gender ambivalent if the same answer (eg, a 1 or a 2) was given to both statements. Gender incongruence was defined as a lower score assigned to the natal sex than to the other sex. Using these definitions, the prevalence of gender incongruence was estimated to be 0.7% for AMAB and 0.6% for AFAB. The corresponding estimates for gender ambivalence among AMAB and AFAB were even higher: 2.2% and 1.9%, respectively.

A study of Taiwanese university students conducted interviews with 5010 participants using the Adult Self-Report Inventory-4 instrument.[45] Self-reported "gender dysphoria" was determined based on a response to the statement "I wish I was the opposite sex." Responses "often" and "very often" were interpreted as evidence of gender dysphoria. The use of this rather loose definition produced high estimated proportions of TGNC people: 7% for AFAB and 1.9% for AMAB.

A recent population-based study evaluated proportion of TGNC people among 50,157 adults residing in Stockholm County, Sweden.[44] The numerator was determined by asking "I would like hormones or surgery to be more like someone of a different sex." Two additional items were designed to identify individuals experiencing gender incongruence: "I feel like someone of a different sex," and "I would like to live as or be treated as someone of a different sex." Responses to each item followed a four-point Likert scale. Using weighting to account for stratified sampling design, the authors reported that the desire for hormone therapy or gender-affirming surgery was reported by 0.5% of participants. Participants who expressed feeling like someone of a different sex and those who wanted to live or be treated as a person of another sex constituted 2.3% and 2.8% of the total sample, respectively.

PROPORTIONS OF CHILDREN AND ADOLESCENTS WITH SELF-REPORTED TRANSGENDER AND GENDER NONCONFORMING IDENTITY

The literature on the proportion of TGNC youth (persons younger than 19 years of age) in the general population is sparse. Four recent studies examined this question by conducting surveys among school children (**Table 4**).[46–49]

Almeida and colleagues[46] used data from the 2006 survey of 9th to 12th grade students in Boston public schools. The survey participants were asked whether they considered themselves transgender (yes, no, do not know), although the precise definition of "transgender" is not given." Of the 1032 complete surveys administered at 18 schools, 17 (1.6%) indicated that the respondents self-identified as transgender. Eleven of the 17 transgender adolescents reported "female as their sex"; this presumably corresponds to the AMAB/AFAB ratio of 1.8:1.

A 2012 national cross-sectional survey in New Zealand collected information on TGNC status among 8166 high school students.[47] The numerator was based on the responses to the question "Do you think you are transgender? This is a girl who feels like she should have been a boy, or a boy who feels like he should have been a girl (eg, Trans, Queen, Fa'faffine, Whakawahine, Tangata ira Tane, Genderqueer)?" The question about TGNC status was preceded by the question "What sex are you?" (with binary response options). A total of 96 students (1.2%) self-identified as TGNC, and 202 (2.5%) reported they were not sure. The AMAB/AFAB ratio for TGNC participants was 1:1.2 and the corresponding estimates for those who responded not sure was 1:1.5. Only about one-third of TGNC participants reported having disclosed their TGNC status.

The most recent of the available publications reported the results of the 2016 survey conducted among 9th and 11th grade students in Minnesota.[48] The data included information on 80,929 survey respondents; of those 2198 students (2.7%) reported being TGNC with AMAB/AFAB ratio of 1:2. The proportions of TGNC adolescents were higher among racial/ethnic minorities, but similar in metropolitan and nonmetropolitan areas of the state.

Only one study examined the proportion of TGNC children in the younger age group. Shields and colleagues[49] analyzed the data from a 2011 survey that included 2730 students (grades 6–8) across 22 public middle schools in San Francisco. Thirty-three children self-identified as TGNC based on the question, "What is your gender?" with the response options "female, male, or transgender." The resulting overall proportion of TGNC survey respondents was 1.3%; however, the results by AMAB/AFAB status were not provided.

PROPORTIONS OF PEOPLE REQUESTING LEGAL NAME OR GENDER CHANGES

Three studies calculated proportions of people who applied for or underwent administrative sex or name change. Two of these studies were conducted in Germany, and one used data from New Zealand.

Weitze and Osburg[50] relied on the 1981 German Transsexuals' Act, which allowed applicants to change their name or documented gender. Within 10 years following implementation of the law, the courts issued 683 decrees on first-name changes and 733 rulings on legal affirmation of gender identity. These rulings involved 1199 individuals, of whom 1047 received approval. Based on the adult population of West Germany before reunification, the proportion of individuals who sought change of their legal record was estimated at 2.1/100,000. The AMAB to AFAB ratio of applicants was approximately 3:1. A more recent report extended the work of Weitze and Osberg by evaluating changes in legal sex status between 1991 and 2000 in all of Germany.[51]

Table 4
Number and population proportion of children and adolescents who self-reported transgender identity and gender nonconformity

Reference	Location; Time Period	Case Definition	Source of Numerator	Numerator Total	AMAB	AFAB	Size of Denominator	Proportion (per 100,000) Total	AMAB	AFAB	Ratio AMAB/AFAB
Almeida et al,[46] 2009	Boston, Massachusetts, 2006	Self-identity as transgender	Boston Youth Survey data	17	11	6	1032	1600			
Clark et al,[47] 2014	New Zealand, 2012	Self-identity as transgender Not sure of gender identity	National survey of secondary school students	96 202	44 82	52 120	8164 (3669 males, 4495 females)	1176 2474	1157 2235	1199 2670	1:1 1:1.2
Eisenberg et al,[48] 2017	Minnesota, 2016	Self-identity as transgender	Minnesota Student Survey	2198			80,929	2700	1700	3600	1:2
Shields et al,[49] 2013	United States, 2011	Self-identity as transgender	Youth Risk Behavior Survey of San Francisco middle schools	33			2701	1300			

The overall proportion of individuals requesting the change was 3.88 per 100,000, using the German population in 2000 as the denominator. The corresponding proportions for AMAB and AFAB were reported to be 4.95 per 100,000 and 2.87 per 100,000, respectively.

In New Zealand, individuals may request a change of their gender marker from "M" or "F" to "X." To determine the frequency of this change, Veale[52] contacted the New Zealand Department of Internal Affairs Passport Office in 2008. A total of 385 such changes were identified. Given the number of passport holders in New Zealand, the proportion of TGNC individuals was calculated as 16 per 100,000 overall, 27 per 100,000 for AMAB, and 4.4 per 100,000 for AFAB.

EVALUATION OF TEMPORAL CHANGES

Virtually all studies evaluating secular trends reported dramatic increases in the numbers (and therefore the population proportions) of TGNC people in recent decades. These observations are confirmed independently regardless of the geographic area of interest, TGNC definition, or statistical methodology. For example, frequency of requests to undergo gender-affirming surgery or hormone therapy were reported to increase between 1960 and 2010 in Sweden,[15] between 1975 and 1992 in the Netherlands,[53] and between 1999 and 2006 in Serbia.[13] Similarly, the proportions of people with documented TGNC status in medical records increased between 1975 and 2015 in the Netherlands,[30] between 2007 and 2015 in Spain,[29] and between 2002 and 2014 across various health systems in the United States.[34,36]

The temporal changes in the proportion of people who self-identify as TGNC are also evident. For example, Meerwijk and Sevelius[2] summarized data from five different population-based surveys that collect data on TGNC identity in the United States. Although the data were limited to the recent years (2007–2015), a meta-regression analysis demonstrated that the proportion of TGNC respondents increased on average 0.026% per year.[2]

Another notable phenomenon is the temporal change in age of presentation. For example, a recent study from Denmark reported that the median age at the time of gender-affirming surgery decreased from 40 years in 1994 to 27 years in 2015.[54] Similar observations were reported more recently with respect to the temporal changes in the median age of the first TGNC-related clinic visit in the Netherlands.[30]

The ratio of AFAB/AMAB also seems to be undergoing transition. In a previously cited study of TGNC people enrolled in Kaiser Permanente the composition of the TGNC population also changed over time.[36] Whereas in 2006 the AMAB/AFAB ratio among TGNC health plan members was approximately 1.7:1, in 2014 the same ratio was 1:1.

The temporal change in the AMAB/AFAB ratio may be especially pronounced among TGNC youth. Two groups of researchers in Canada and in the Netherlands compared data from their respective specialized gender identity clinics for the most recent time period (2006–2013) versus earlier years.[55] At both study sites, there was a notable switch in the AMAB/AFAB ratio. In Canada the ratio changed approximately 1.4:1 in the earlier time period to 1:1.7 in the later period. The changes in the Netherlands were reported to be in the same direction.

A similarly designed study conducted in the United Kingdom reported evidence that the AMAB/AFAB ratio among adolescents changed from 1.6:1 in 2009 to 1:2.5 in 2016. The corresponding ratios for children (younger than 12 years of age) changed from 5:1 to approximately 1:1.[56] In an expanded analysis of the same data covering the period from 2000 to 2017, the results were generally the same.[57]

DISCUSSION

The current literature on the number and proportion of TGNC people is highly heterogeneous. Whereas in most studies focusing on individuals who seek or receive TGNC-related care at specialized institutions, the estimates of interest generally ranged between 1 and 30 per 100,000 individuals, self-reported TGNC identity was found to be orders of magnitude more frequent. The reported proportions of people self-identified as TGNC ranged from 100 to 2000 per 100,000 or 0.1% to 2% among adults. The corresponding range among schoolchildren was 1.3% to 2.7%. One study reported an even higher proportion of almost 5%,[45] but there is a good reason to suspect that the specific survey item ("I wish I was the opposite sex") used in that study may have resulted in an inflated estimate.

In addition to differences in definitions, other sources of heterogeneity across reported results may include diverse cultural and legal population-specific contexts and a wide range of time periods covered in different studies. With respect to the former, the magnitude of the reported proportions may depend on how TGNC people are perceived and treated in a society. With respect to the latter, the reported inconsistencies of findings over time are likely attributable to the increasing likelihood of acknowledging and disclosing one's TGNC status.

Proportion, by definition, is a ratio in which all observations in the numerator arise from a predefined denominator. With this definition in mind, it is important to acknowledge that most studies included in this review first assessed the number of patients seen at a particular clinical center and then divided that number by an approximated population size. Such an approach is unlikely to produce an accurate estimate because the numerator and the denominator are ascertained without a defined sampling frame and are both subject to error. These methodologic shortcomings have been discussed previously, and it is encouraging that several of the recently published studies were able to use more formal statistical methodology.[35,36,41,44]

In summary, it is clear that people who identify as TGNC represent a sizable proportion of the general population. Based on the credible evidence available to date, this proportion currently ranges from 0.1% to 2.7%, depending on the inclusion criteria, age of participants, and geographic location. By contrast, clinic-based studies seem to capture only a small subset of the TGNC population. It is also clear that TGNC population is undergoing rapid changes in terms of its size and in terms of its demographic characteristics, such as age of "coming out," and AMAB/AFAB ratio. Accurate estimates of the proportion, distribution, and composition of the TGNC population depend on the availability of systematically collected high-quality data. Far more accurate and precise estimates should become available when population censuses begin collecting data on sex assigned at birth and gender identity, including nonbinary categories.

REFERENCES

1. Deutsch MB. Making it count: improving estimates of the size of transgender and gender nonconforming populations. LGBT Health 2016;3(3):181–5.
2. Meerwijk EL, Sevelius JM. Transgender population size in the United States: a meta-regression of population-based probability samples. Am J Public Health 2017;107(2):e1–8.
3. Coleman E, Bockting WO, Botzer M, et al. Standards of care for the health of transsexual, transgender, and gender-nonconforming people, version 7. Int J Transgend 2012;13(4):165–232.

4. Meier SC, Labuski CM. The demographics of the transgender population. In: International handbook on the demography of sexuality. Springer Dodrecht, Netherlands; 2013. p. 289–327.

5. Arcelus J, Bouman WP, Van Den Noortgate W, et al. Systematic review and meta-analysis of prevalence studies in transsexualism. Eur Psychiatry 2015;30(6): 807–15.

6. Collin L, Reisner SL, Tangpricha V, et al. Prevalence of transgender depends on the "case" definition: a systematic review. J Sex Med 2016;13(4):613–26.

7. Adams N, Pearce R, Veale J, et al. Guidance and ethical considerations for undertaking transgender health research and institutional review boards adjudicating this research. Transgend Health 2017;2(1):165–75.

8. Bouman WP, Schwend AS, Motmans J, et al. Language and trans health. Int J Transgend 2017;18(1):1–6.

9. Rothman KJ, Greenland S. Modern epidemiology. Philadelphia: Lippincott Williams and Wilkins; 1998.

10. Caldarera A, Pfäfflin F. Transsexualism and sex reassignment surgery in Italy. Int J Transgend 2011;13(1):26–36.

11. De Cuypere G, Vanhemelrijck M, Michel A, et al. Prevalence and demography of transsexualism in Belgium. Eur Psychiatry 2007;22(3):137–41.

12. Tsoi WF. The prevalence of transsexualism in Singapore. Acta Psychiatr Scand 1988;78(4):501–4.

13. Vujovic S, Popovic S, Sbutega-Milosevic G, et al. Transsexualism in Serbia: a twenty-year follow-up study. J Sex Med 2009;6(4):1018–23.

14. Pauly IB. The current status of the change of sex operation. J Nerv Ment Dis 1968; 147(5):460–71.

15. Dhejne C, Oberg K, Arver S, et al. An analysis of all applications for sex reassignment surgery in Sweden, 1960-2010: prevalence, incidence, and regrets. Arch Sex Behav 2014;43(8):1535–45.

16. Esteva de Antonio I, Gomez-Gil E, Almaraz MC, et al. Organization of Healthcare for transsexual persons in the Spanish National Health System. Gac Sanit 2012; 26(3):203–9 [in Spanish].

17. Eklund PL, Gooren LJ, Bezemer PD. Prevalence of transsexualism in the Netherlands. Br J Psychiatry 1988;152:638–40.

18. Bakker A, van Kesteren PJ, Gooren LJ, et al. The prevalence of transsexualism in the Netherlands. Acta Psychiatr Scand 1993;87(4):237–8.

19. Hoenig J, Kenna JC. The prevalence of transsexualism in England and Wales. Br J Psychiatry 1974;124(579):181–90.

20. Esteva I, Gonzalo M, Yahyaoui R, et al. Epidemiología De La Transexualidad En Andalucía, Atención Especial Al Grupo De Adolescentes. C Med Psicosom 2006; 78:65–70.

21. Gómez Gil E, Trilla Garcia A, Godas Sieso T, et al. Estimation of prevalence, incidence and sex ratio of transsexualism in Catalonia according to health care demand. Actas Esp Psiquiatr 2006;34(5):295–302 [in Spanish].

22. Okabe N, Sato T, Matsumoto Y, et al. Clinical characteristics of patients with gender identity disorder at a Japanese Gender Identity Disorder Clinic. Psychiatry Res 2008;157(1):315–8.

23. Baba T, Endo T, Ikeda K, et al. Distinctive features of female-to-male transsexualism and prevalence of gender identity disorder in Japan. J Sex Med 2011; 8(6):1686–93.

24. Ahmadzad-Asl M, Jalali A-H, Alavi K, et al. The epidemiology of transsexualism in Iran. J Gay Lesbian Ment Health 2010;15(1):83–93.

25. Judge C, O'Donovan C, Callaghan G, et al. Gender dysphoria: prevalence and co-morbidities in an Irish adult population. Front Endocrinol (Lausanne) 2014; 5:87.

26. Wålinder J. Transsexualism: definition, prevalence sex distribution. Acta Psychiatr Scand 1968;43(S203):255–8.

27. Ross MW, Walinder J, Lundstrom B, et al. Cross-cultural approaches to transsexualism. a comparison between Sweden and Australia. Acta Psychiatr Scand 1981;63(1):75–82.

28. Wilson P, Sharp C, Carr S. The prevalence of gender dysphoria in Scotland: a primary care study. Br J Gen Pract 1999;49(449):991–2.

29. Becerra-Fernández A, Rodriguez-Molina JM, Asenjo-Araque N, et al. Prevalence, incidence, and sex ratio of transsexualism in the autonomous region of Madrid (Spain) according to healthcare demand. Arch Sex Behav 2017;46(5):1307–12.

30. Wiepjes CM, Nota NM, de Blok CJM, et al. The Amsterdam Cohort of Gender Dysphoria Study (1972-2015): trends in prevalence, treatment, and regrets. J Sex Med 2018;15(4):582–90.

31. O'Gorman EC. A retrospective study of epidemiological and clinical aspects of 28 transsexual patients. Arch Sex Behav 1982;11(3):231–6.

32. Hwu HG, Yeh EK, Chang LY. Prevalence of psychiatric disorders in Taiwan defined by the Chinese diagnostic interview schedule. Acta Psychiatr Scand 1989;79(2):136–47.

33. Stefansson JG, Lindal E, Bjornsson JK, et al. Lifetime prevalence of specific mental disorders among people born in Iceland in 1931. Acta Psychiatr Scand 1991;84(2):142–9.

34. Blosnich JR, Brown GR, Shipherd Phd JC, et al. Prevalence of gender identity disorder and suicide risk among transgender veterans utilizing Veterans Health Administration Care. Am J Public Health 2013;103(10):e27–32.

35. Kauth MR, Shipherd JC, Lindsay J, et al. Access to care for transgender veterans in the Veterans Health Administration: 2006-2013. Am J Public Health 2014; 104(Suppl 4):S532–4.

36. Quinn VP, Nash R, Hunkeler E, et al. Cohort profile: study of transition, outcomes and gender (Strong) to assess health status of transgender people. BMJ Open 2017;7(12):e018121.

37. Conron KJ, Scott G, Stowell GS, et al. Transgender health in Massachusetts: results from a household probability sample of adults. Am J Public Health 2012; 102(1):118–22.

38. Crissman HP, Berger MB, Graham LF, et al. Transgender demographics: a household probability sample of US adults, 2014. Am J Public Health 2017;107(2): 213–5.

39. Flores A, Herman J, Gates G, et al. How many adults identify as transgender in the United States. Los Angeles (CA): The Williams Insitute, UCLA School of Law; 2016.

40. Gates GJ. How many people are lesbian, gay, bisexual and transgender? Los Angeles (CA): Williams Institute, University of California, Los Angeles School of Law; 2011.

41. Reisner SL, Conron KJ, Tardiff LA, et al. Monitoring the health of transgender and other gender minority populations: validity of natal sex and gender identity survey items in a U.S. National Cohort of Young Adults. BMC Public Health 2014;14:1224.

42. Kuyper L, Wijsen C. Gender identities and gender dysphoria in the Netherlands. Arch Sex Behav 2014;43(2):377–85.

43. Van Caenegem E, Wierckx K, Elaut E, et al. Prevalence of gender nonconformity in Flanders, Belgium. Arch Sex Behav 2015;44(5):1281–7.
44. Ahs JW, Dhejne C, Magnusson C, et al. Proportion of adults in the general population of Stockholm County who want gender-affirming medical treatment. PLoS One 2018;13(10):e0204606.
45. Lai MC, Chiu YN, Gadow KD, et al. Correlates of gender dysphoria in Taiwanese University Students. Arch Sex Behav 2010;39(6):1415–28.
46. Almeida J, Johnson RM, Corliss HL, et al. Emotional distress among LGBT youth: the influence of perceived discrimination based on sexual orientation. J Youth Adolesc 2009;38(7):1001–14.
47. Clark TC, Lucassen MF, Bullen P, et al. The health and well-being of transgender high school students: results from the New Zealand adolescent health survey (Youth'12). J Adolesc Health 2014;55(1):93–9.
48. Eisenberg ME, Gower AL, McMorris BJ, et al. Risk and protective factors in the lives of transgender/gender nonconforming adolescents. J Adolesc Health 2017;61(4):521–6.
49. Shields JP, Cohen R, Glassman JR, et al. Estimating population size and demographic characteristics of lesbian, gay, bisexual, and transgender youth in middle school. J Adolesc Health 2013;52(2):248–50.
50. Weitze C, Osburg S. Transsexualism in Germany: empirical data on epidemiology and application of the German transsexuals' act during its first ten years. Arch Sex Behav 1996;25(4):409–25.
51. Meyer zu Hoerge SP. Inzidenz Und Geschlechterverhaltnis Der Transsexualitat Anhand Der Bundesweit Getroffenen Entscheidungen Nach Dem Transsexuellengesetz in Der Zeit Von 1991 Bis 2000. Kiel (Germany): Christia-Albrechts-Universitat zu Kiel; 2010.
52. Veale JF. Prevalence of transsexualism among New Zealand passport holders. Aus N Z J Psychiatry 2008;42(10):887–9.
53. van Kesteren PJ, Gooren LJ, Megens JA. An epidemiological and demographic study of transsexuals in the Netherlands. Arch Sex Behav 1996;25(6):589–600.
54. Aydin D, Buk LJ, Partoft S, et al. Transgender surgery in Denmark from 1994 to 2015: 20-year follow-up study. J Sex Med 2016;13(4):720–5.
55. Aitken M, Steensma TD, Blanchard R, et al. Evidence for an altered sex ratio in clinic-referred adolescents with gender dysphoria. J Sex Med 2015;12(3):756–63.
56. de Graaf NM, Giovanardi G, Zitz C, et al. Sex ratio in children and adolescents referred to the gender identity development service in the UK (2009-2016). Arch Sex Behav 2018;47(5):1301–4.
57. de Graaf NM, Carmichael P, Steensma TD, et al. Evidence for a change in the sex ratio of children referred for gender dysphoria: data from the gender identity development service in London (2000-2017). J Sex Med 2018;15(10):1381–3.

Etiology of Gender Identity

Sira Korpaisarn, MD[a,*], Joshua D. Safer, MD[b]

KEYWORDS

- Gender identity • Gender expression • Transgender • Etiology

KEY POINTS

- There are no data to suggest that gender identity is manipulated by external forces.
- Prenatal androgen exposure may influence gender identity and gender expression in some individuals.
- No specific genetic locus or neuroanatomic region is consistently identified as a cause of gender identity.

INTRODUCTION

Transgender persons are individuals who have gender identity incongruent with sex designated at birth. Numerous terms in the transgender medical field carry overlapped definitions, which cause confusion among health care providers involved in transgender care. Magnus Hirschfeld first introduced the word "transvestite" in 1910s referring to individuals who derive pleasure from dressing in clothes of the other sex. Later, in 1940s David Cauldwell, a US psychiatrist, used the word "transsexual" referring to individuals who have completed transgender medical and surgical interventions.[1] In 1967 the term transsexual became widespread because of a publication by Harry Benjamin,[2] a pioneer in the transgender medical field.

In the past, being transgender was defined as a mental health concern and was categorized as such by the World Health Organization in the International Classification of Diseases-10. The recognition of the biologic underpinnings to gender identity has resulted in a major framework shift. Indeed, the latest International Classification of Diseases-11, launched in 2018, changed the term to "gender incongruence" and reclassified it under conditions related to sexual health.[3]

The term gender dysphoria, which has been used interchangeably with being transgender, more accurately describes distress related to the gender incongruence noted previously. Many transgender individuals suffer no dysphoria but still

Disclosure Statement: The authors have nothing to disclose.
[a] Section of Endocrinology, Diabetes, Nutrition and Weight Management, Boston Medical Center, Boston University School of Medicine, 720 Harrison Avenue, 8th Floor, Suite 8100, Boston, MA 02118, USA; [b] Center for Transgender Medicine and Surgery, Mount Sinai Health System, Icahn School of Medicine at Mount Sinai, 275 7th Avenue, Suite 1505, New York, NY 10001, USA
* Corresponding author.
E-mail address: sira.korpaisarn@bmc.org

require medical and/or surgical interventions to align their bodies with their gender identities. For those transgender individuals with a diagnosis of gender dysphoria, it is not clear that a separate diagnostic term is required beyond the existing dysphoria diagnosis in the Diagnostic and Statistical Manual of Mental Disorders (with no modifier), although many payers still insist on "gender dysphoria" as a diagnostic term.

The Endocrine Society launched the most recent guidelines for treatment of transgender persons in 2017.[4] The guideline defines several terms commonly used in transgender care. Gender identity refers to one's internal, deeply held sense of gender. For transgender people, gender identity does not match their sex designated at birth. Gender expression is defined as external manifestations of gender, expressed through one's name, pronouns, clothing, haircut, behavior, voice, or body characteristics. Sexual orientation is used to describe an individual's physical and emotional attraction to another person.

Neither gender identity nor gender expression are confined strictly to male or female in a binary fashion. Although most people report a simple binary gender identity, some report gender identities that lie between all male and all female, or even neither.[5] A large Dutch survey among 8064 people revealed that 3.2% to 4.6% of individuals reported an ambivalent gender identity.[5] The nonbinary population may present some challenge for health care providers in some settings because there is no available standard of care for this particular population.

This article reviews the current literature discussing the factors contributing to gender identity.

ETIOLOGY OF GENDER IDENTITY

Several factors are connected to the development of gender identity. Specific biologic factors include yet to be further elucidated biologic explanations, prenatal androgen exposure, and neuroanatomy.

Failure to Manipulate Gender Identity Subsequent to Birth

Attempts to change gender identity external forces have proved unsuccessful. Meyer-Bahlburg[6] reviewed the outcome of gender assignment to female of 46, XY newborns with intersex conditions from nonhormonal causes presumed to have normal male prenatal hormonal milieu. Conditions included penile agenesis, cloacal exstrophy of the bladder, and penile ablation.[6] Only 47% of female-raised patients remained living as females without gender dysphoria in adulthood. Furthermore, among a cohort of 14 XY individuals with cloacal exstrophy who underwent female sex assignment socially, legally, and surgically, all individuals who knew their medical history (57%) reported male gender identity.[7]

Association of Androgen Exposure on Gender Identity and Gender Expression

Early animal evidence suggested that pregnant guinea pigs with testosterone exposure had female offspring with more malelike behavior in adulthood and less female-like behavior.[8] This study led to several animal studies reproducing the concept of androgen exposure prenatally resulting in male-type behavior among females.[9]

Among human females with virilizing congenital adrenal hyperplasia, a disproportionate preference for male-typical play in childhood has been reported.[10] Similarly, the prevalence of gender dysphoria among females with virilizing congenital adrenal hyperplasia is significantly higher (3%) than what is seen in the population in general (0.6%).[11,12]

In contrast, XY-individuals with complete androgen insensitivity syndrome (CAIS) usually have female gender identity.[13,14] There are a few case reports of male gender identity among females with CAIS raised as female.[15,16]

Individuals with 5-α-reductase deficiency often have ambiguous genitalia at birth because of the lack of dihydrotestosterone and may be raised as female. However, pubertal virilization occurs because testosterone synthesis and peripheral action are intact. Up to 63% of such individuals change gender expression from female to male at puberty.[17] A study in 18 XY individuals with 5- α-reductase deficiency reared as female suggested that 17 of 18 eventually reported male gender identity in puberty.[18] Although gender expression changed it is not clear there was any shift in gender identity.

Endogenous Biology

Gender identity is not chromosomal. For example, XY-individuals with CAIS commonly have female gender identity.[13,14] However, there is evidence for a significant endogenous biologic component underlying gender identity. A British study among 4426 female twins claimed an 11% genetic component for gender identity in adults.[19] An Australian study of 4901 twins, male and female, reported the authors' calculation of familial factors acting on gender identity to range from 24% to 31%.[20] In a review of case reports of transgender individuals with twins, 39% of monozygotic twins were concordant with transgender identity but none of the dizygotic twins were concordant with transgender identity.[21] Although the methodology is flawed, others have constructed algorithms that are claimed as evidence of a genetic element underlying gender identity and/or gender dysphoria.[22,23]

Several attempts have been made to associate specific gene signatures with transgender identity. The CYP17 genes, encoding for 17- α-hydroxylase, along with the RYR3 gene related to calcium homeostasis have been proposed to be associated with transmasculine identity.[24–26]

Neuroanatomy

Several neuroanatomic structures may differ between men and women. For example, there are reports that total brain volume and amygdala are larger in men, whereas cortical brain and hippocampus are greater in women.[27] A potential neuroanatomic association between gender identity and the bed nucleus of the stria terminalis (BST) in hypothalamus has been proposed. BST is a part of limbic system that plays a role in sexual behavior in animal studies.[28] A postmortem study revealed that transgender women had decreased BST neurons in a pattern similar to that of the nontransgender women and that transgender men had increased BST neurons.[28,29] The findings were not the result of sex hormone alteration in adulthood but rather established in early brain development. The interstitial nucleus of the anterior hypothalamus 3 (INAH3) is another area of the brain where some report a difference between men and women. INAH3 is a sexually dimorphic hypothalamic nucleus with a possible connection to the BST along with other brain nuclei associated with gender identity and sexual behavior. There is a report of transgender individuals with volume of INAH3 matching gender identity.[30]

SUMMARY

Development of gender identity and gender expression are multidimensional process involving interaction among numerous factors. Prenatal androgen exposure may play a role for some individuals. Studies claiming possible genetic loci related to transmasculine

Table 1
Studies with regard to factors associated with gender identity/gender expression

Authors/y	Study Design	N/Subjects	Main Findings
Androgen exposure			
Dessens et al,[12] 2005	Case series	283/46, XX with CAH	2.8% prevalence of gender dysphoria among females with virilizing CAH.
Hines et al,[10] 2004	Case-control	25/CAH	Women with CAH recalled significantly more male-typical play behavior.
Hines et al,[14] 2003	Case-control	22/46, XY with CAIS	No significant differences in core gender identity or gender role behavior compared with control females.
Wisniewski et al,[13] 2000	Case series	14/46, XY with CAIS	All were satisfied with having been raised as females.
Cohen-Kettenis,[17] 2005	Case series	99/46, XY with 5α-reductase-deficiency	63% changed gender expression from female to male at puberty.
Imperato-McGinley et al,[18] 1979	Case series	33/46, XY with 5α-reductase-deficiency	17 of 18 female-raised patients later reported a male-gender identity and 16 of 18 to a male-gender role.
Heritable genetic components			
Burri et al,[19] 2011	Case-control	4426/female twins	An algorithm purporting gender identity is 11% under genetic influence.
Bailey et al,[20] 2000	Case-control	4901/twins	An algorithm purporting gender identity is 24%–31% under genetic influence.
Sasaki et al,[23] 2016	Case-control	3302/twin pairs	An algorithm purporting gender dysphoria is 11% under genetic influence.
Heylens et al,[21] 2012	Case-control	44/twins	39% of monozygotic twins were concordant with transgender identity but none of the dizygotic twins were concordant with transgender identity.
Coolidge et al,[22] 2002	Case-control	314/twins	An algorithm purporting gender dysphoria is 62% under genetic influence.
Sex hormone–related genes			
Yang et al,[26] 2017	Case-control	13/transgender persons	Mutations in RYR3 gene were more prevalent in transgender males but none in control subjects.
Fernández et al,[24] 2015	Case-control	293/transgender persons	The frequency of A2 allele of the CYP17 MspA1 polymorphism was significantly higher in transgender males.

Bentz et al,[25] 2008	Case-control	151/transgender persons	CYP17–34 T > C SNP allele frequencies were significantly different between transgender male individuals and nontransgender female control subjects.
Fernández et al,[31] 2014	Case-control	273/transgender males	The repeat length polymorphism of the ERβ gene was significantly higher in transgender males compared with nontransgender females.
Henningsson et al,[32] 2005	Case-control	29/transgender females	The mean length of the ERβ repeat polymorphism was different in transgender females compared with nontransgender males.
Hare et al,[33] 2009	Case-control	258/transgender females	The CAG repeat lengths in the AR gene were significantly longer in transgender females relative to nontransgender males.
Fernández et al,[34] 2014	Case-control	442/transgender females	No evidence of association between either ERβ, AR, or aromatase genes and transgender females.
Ujike et al,[35] 2009	Case-control	242/transgender persons	No significant difference in genotypic distribution of AR, ERα, ERβ, aromatase or progesterone receptor between transgender persons and nontransgender persons.
Neuroanatomy			
Kruijver et al,[29] 2000	Postmortem	7/brains of transgender persons	Transgender females had fewer neurons in BST similar to nontransgender females. Transgender males had more BST neurons similar to nontransgender males.
Zhou et al,[28] 1995	Postmortem	6/brains of transgender females	Transgender females had decreased staining of BST similar to nontransgender females.
Garcia-Falgueras & Swaab,[30] 2008	Postmortem	12/brains of transgender persons	Transgender females had fewer neurons and decreased volume in INAH3 similar to nontransgender females. Transgender males had more neurons and increased volume in INAH3 similar to nontransgender males.
Failure to manipulate gender identity by external forces			
Meyer-Bahlburg,[6] 2005	Case series	388/46, XY with severe genital abnormalities	Only 47% of female-raised patients were living as females without gender dysphoria in adulthood. There was an increased risk of later patient-initiated gender reassignment to male despite the original female assignment.
Reiner & Gearhart,[7] 2004	Case series	16/46, XY with cloacal-exstrophy	57% of female-raised patients later reported male gender identity including all who knew their medical histories as of the time the paper was written.

Abbreviations: AR, androgen receptor; BST, the bed nucleus of the stria terminalis; CAH, congenital adrenal hyperplasia; CAIS, complete androgen insensitivity syndrome; ER, estrogen receptor; INAH3, the interstitial nucleus of the anterior hypothalamus 3; SNP, single-nucleotide polymorphisms.

identity include those for 17- α-hydroxylase (CYP17) genes, RYR3 gene, and ERβ genes (**Table 1**). Two neuroanatomic regions, BST and INAH3, have been associated with gender identity. Although mechanisms have not been demonstrated, gender identity seems a durable, biologic phenomenon that is not shaped by external forces. No environmental influence on gender identity has been identified to date.

REFERENCES

1. Meyerowitz JJ. How sex changed: A history of transsexuality in the United States. Cambridge (MA): Harvard University Press; 2009.
2. Benjamin H. The transsexual phenomenon. Trans N Y Acad Sci 1967;29(4): 428–30.
3. World Health Organization. WHO releases new International Classification of Diseases (ICD 11). Available at: http://www.who.int/news-room/detail/18-06-2018-who-releases-new-international-classification-of-diseases-(icd-11). Accessed October 1, 2018.
4. Hembree WC, Cohen-Kettenis PT, Gooren L, et al. Endocrine treatment of gender-dysphoric/gender-incongruent persons: an Endocrine Society clinical practice guideline. J Clin Endocrinol Metab 2017;102(11):3869–903.
5. Kuyper L, Wijsen C. Gender identities and gender dysphoria in the Netherlands. Arch Sex Behav 2014;43(2):377–85.
6. Meyer-Bahlburg HFL. Gender identity outcome in female-raised 46,XY persons with penile agenesis, cloacal exstrophy of the bladder, or penile ablation. Arch Sex Behav 2005;34(4):423–38.
7. Reiner WG, Gearhart JP. Discordant sexual identity in some genetic males with cloacal exstrophy assigned to female sex at birth. N Engl J Med 2004;350(4):333–41.
8. Phoenix CH, Goy RW, Gerall AA, et al. Organizing action of prenatally administered testosterone propionate on the tissues mediating mating behavior in the female guinea pig. Endocrinology 1959;65:369–82.
9. Arnold AP, McCarthy MM. Sexual differentiation of the brain and behavior: a primer. In: Pfaff DW, Volkow ND, editors. Neuroscience in the 21st century. New York: Springer; 2016. p. 2139–68.
10. Hines M, Brook C, Conway GS. Androgen and psychosexual development: core gender identity, sexual orientation and recalled childhood gender role behavior in women and men with congenital adrenal hyperplasia (CAH). J Sex Res 2004; 41(1):75–81.
11. Flores AR, Herman J, Gates GJ, et al. How many adults identify as transgender in the United States? Los Angeles (CA): The Williams Institute; 2016. Available at: https://escholarship.org/uc/item/2kg9x2rk.
12. Dessens AB, Slijper FME, Drop SLS. Gender dysphoria and gender change in chromosomal females with congenital adrenal hyperplasia. Arch Sex Behav 2005;34(4):389–97.
13. Wisniewski AB, Migeon CJ, Meyer-Bahlburg HF, et al. Complete androgen insensitivity syndrome: long-term medical, surgical, and psychosexual outcome. J Clin Endocrinol Metab 2000;85(8):2664–9.
14. Hines M, Ahmed SF, Hughes IA. Psychological outcomes and gender-related development in complete androgen insensitivity syndrome. Arch Sex Behav 2003;32(2):93–101.
15. T'Sjoen G, De Cuypere G, Monstrey S, et al. Male gender identity in complete androgen insensitivity syndrome. Arch Sex Behav 2011;40(3):635–8.

16. Kulshreshtha B, Philibert P, Eunice M, et al. Apparent male gender identity in a patient with complete androgen insensitivity syndrome. Arch Sex Behav 2009; 38(6):873–5.
17. Cohen-Kettenis PT. Gender change in 46,XY persons with 5alpha-reductase-2 deficiency and 17beta-hydroxysteroid dehydrogenase-3 deficiency. Arch Sex Behav 2005;34(4):399–410.
18. Imperato-McGinley J, Peterson RE, Gautier T, et al. Androgens and the evolution of male-gender identity among male pseudohermaphrodites with 5alpha-reductase deficiency. N Engl J Med 1979;300(22):1233–7.
19. Burri A, Cherkas L, Spector T, et al. Genetic and environmental influences on female sexual orientation, childhood gender typicality and adult gender identity. PLoS One 2011;6(7):e21982.
20. Bailey JM, Michael Bailey J, Dunne MP, et al. Genetic and environmental influences on sexual orientation and its correlates in an Australian twin sample. J Pers Soc Psychol 2000;78(3):524–36.
21. Heylens G, De Cuypere G, Zucker KJ, et al. Gender identity disorder in twins: a review of the case report literature. J Sex Med 2012;9(3):751–7.
22. Coolidge FL, Thede LL, Young SE. The heritability of gender identity disorder in a child and adolescent twin sample. Behav Genet 2002;32(4):251–7.
23. Sasaki S, Ozaki K, Yamagata S, et al. Genetic and environmental influences on traits of gender identity disorder: a study of Japanese twins across developmental stages. Arch Sex Behav 2016;45(7):1681–95.
24. Fernández R, Cortés-Cortés J, Esteva I, et al. The CYP17 MspA1 polymorphism and the gender dysphoria. J Sex Med 2015;12(6):1329–33.
25. Bentz E-K, Hefler LA, Kaufmann U, et al. A polymorphism of the CYP17 gene related to sex steroid metabolism is associated with female-to-male but not male-to-female transsexualism. Fertil Steril 2008;90(1):56–9.
26. Yang F, Zhu X-H, Zhang Q, et al. Genomic characteristics of gender dysphoria patients and identification of rare mutations in RYR3 gene. Sci Rep 2017;7(1): 8339.
27. Luders E, Toga AW. Sex differences in brain anatomy. Prog Brain Res 2010;186: 3–12.
28. Zhou JN, Hofman MA, Gooren LJ, et al. A sex difference in the human brain and its relation to transsexuality. Nature 1995;378(6552):68–70.
29. Kruijver FP, Zhou JN, Pool CW, et al. Male-to-female transsexuals have female neuron numbers in a limbic nucleus. J Clin Endocrinol Metab 2000;85(5): 2034–41.
30. Garcia-Falgueras A, Swaab DF. A sex difference in the hypothalamic uncinate nucleus: relationship to gender identity. Brain 2008;131(Pt 12):3132–46.
31. Fernández R, Esteva I, Gómez-Gil E, et al. The (CA)n polymorphism of ERβ gene is associated with FtM transsexualism. J Sex Med 2014;11(3):720–8.
32. Henningsson S, Westberg L, Nilsson S, et al. Sex steroid-related genes and male-to-female transsexualism. Psychoneuroendocrinology 2005;30(7):657–64.
33. Hare L, Bernard P, Sánchez FJ, et al. Androgen receptor repeat length polymorphism associated with male-to-female transsexualism. Biol Psychiatry 2009; 65(1):93–6.
34. Fernández R, Esteva I, Gómez-Gil E, et al. Association study of ERβ, AR, and CYP19A1 genes and MtF transsexualism. J Sex Med 2014;11(12):2986–94.
35. Ujike H, Otani K, Nakatsuka M, et al. Association study of gender identity disorder and sex hormone-related genes. Prog Neuropsychopharmacol Biol Psychiatry 2009;33(7):1241–4.

Hormone Therapy in Children and Adolescents

Jessica Abramowitz, MD

KEYWORDS

- Transgender youth • Pubertal suppression • GnRH analogs
- Gender-affirming hormones

KEY POINTS

- For adolescents with gender dysphoria in early stages of puberty, puberty may be suppressed using gonadotropin-releasing hormone analogs.
- Transgender adolescents may be treated with gender-affirming hormones using estradiol and testosterone for feminization or masculinization if gender dysphoria continues after pubertal suppression.
- Ongoing monitoring is required during pubertal suppression treatment and gender-affirming hormones to monitor for both expected and adverse effects.

INTRODUCTION

Gender identity forms in early childhood and children as young as 2 years to 3 years old are able to identify gender in themselves and others.[1] Gender dysphoria occurs when an individual experiences distress due to a gender identity that differs from the gender assigned at birth, with an associated difficulty in functioning because of this difference.[2] Gender dysphoria can manifest in children as well as adults and there are specific diagnostic criteria included in the *Diagnostic and Statistical Manual of Mental Disorders* (Fifth edition) for this diagnosis in children (**Box 1**).[2] To qualify for this diagnosis, children must meet 6 of the criteria in addition to having distress or impaired functioning lasting for at least 6 months.[2] Gender dysphoria can present at different points in childhood, but for most children it does not persist into adulthood.[3] There has been an overall increasing number of individuals diagnosed with gender dysphoria over the past several years.[4] Following this trend, there have been higher numbers of transgender youth presenting for treatment, and this uptrend in referrals has been noted in multiple pediatric gender clinics.[5–8] In addition, in these clinics, more transgender boys are presenting for care.[9]

The care of transgender children and adolescents requires a multidisciplinary team, including hormone prescribing physicians as well as mental health professionals.[10,11] After psychological evaluation, transgender adolescents may be started on treatment

Disclosure Statement: None.
Division of Endocrinology and Metabolism, Department of Medicine, UT Southwestern Medical Center, 2001 Inwood Road, Dallas, TX 75390, USA
E-mail address: JESSICA.ABRAMOWITZ@UTSOUTHWESTERN.EDU

Endocrinol Metab Clin N Am 48 (2019) 331–339
https://doi.org/10.1016/j.ecl.2019.01.003
0889-8529/19/© 2019 Elsevier Inc. All rights reserved.

Box 1
Diagnostic criteria for gender dysphoria in children

1. A strong desire to be of the other gender or an insistence that one is the other gender
2. A strong preference for wearing clothes typical of the opposite gender
3. A strong preference for cross-gender roles in make-believe play or fantasy play
4. A strong preference for the toys, games or activities stereotypically used or engaged in by the other gender
5. A strong preference for playmates of the other gender
6. A strong rejection of toys, games, and activities typical of one's assigned gender
7. A strong dislike of one's sexual anatomy
8. A strong desire for the physical sex characteristics that match one's experienced gender

---

with either pubertal blockade or gender-affirming hormones to relieve dysphoria and better align their physical features with their gender identity.[10]

PUBERTAL BLOCKADE

Puberty begins with the pulsatile secretion of gonadotropin-releasing hormone (GnRH) from the hypothalamus, which stimulates the release of luteinizing hormone (LH) and follicle-stimulating hormone (FSH) from the pituitary gland. LH and FSH stimulate the ovaries in girls and the testes in boys to secrete estrogen and testosterone, respectively. The presence of circulating testosterone and estradiol leads to the noted physical changes of puberty. The intensity of gender dysphoria in childhood has been linked to its persistence into adolescence.[12,13] Gender dysphoria usually persists for those youth who have intensification of dysphoria with the onset puberty.[3,6,13] Current guidelines for the treatment of gender dysphoria, including the Endocrine Society guidelines and the World Professional Association for Transgender Health Standards of Care, support the treatment of adolescents in early stages of puberty with pubertal blockade.[10,11] Pubertal suppression is typically started at Tanner stage 2:

For girls, breast development:

- Tanner stage 2 = breast and papilla elevated, increased areola diameter

For boys, genital development:

- Tanner stage 2 = penile enlargement, enlarged scrotum, testes 4 mL to 6 mL[10]

Studies of the effects of pubertal suppression using GnRH analogs have shown improved psychosocial functioning for transgender youth.[14,15] In a cohort of 70 children with gender dysphoria who were treated with pubertal suppression, there was a decrease in behavioral and emotional issues as well as depression. In addition, none of the treated individuals discontinued treatment and all proceeded with gender-affirming hormonal treatment.[15] Suppression of puberty allows more time for gender exploration and experience in the affirmed gender role before deciding to let puberty of the gender assigned at birth proceed or to start gender-affirming hormones.[10,11] If started in early puberty, suppression of pubertal hormones allows for better cosmetic outcomes for transgender individuals who subsequently are treated with gender-affirming hormones because the irreversible physical changes of puberty will not occur **(Table 1)**.[6,10]

Table 1 Risks and benefits of pubertal suppression	
Risks	**Benefits**
Effects on bone density	Time for gender exploration
Compromised fertility	Improved cosmetic outcomes
Unknown effects on brain development	Fully reversible
	Improved psychological functioning

GnRH analogs are the preferred agent for suppression of puberty.[10] GnRH analogs work to suppress the pituitary gonadal axis by suppressing LH and FSH and their effect on the gonads and sex hormone production and have been used for the suppression of puberty in children with precocious puberty,[16] and their use has been safe and effective.[17] Commonly used agents include goserelin, leuprolide, or histrelin and are administered subcutaneously once monthly or once every 3 months or as a longer-term implant. This protocol is based on studies published from the Netherlands in which transgender youth were treated with GnRH analogs for pubertal suppression.[14,15] GnRH analogs have been shown to effectively suppress puberty in the transgender population with decreased gonadotropin and sex steroid levels, with no significant effect on kidney or liver function.[18]

Prior to the initiation of GnRH analogs, the pediatric endocrinologist should confirm that puberty has started and that there is an indication for GnRH analog treatment, and the mental health professional should verify the diagnosis of gender dysphoria and the following criteria:

- Dysphoria is long lasting and persistent.
- The gender dysphoria is worsened by puberty
- Medical, psychological, or social concerns are addressed.
- Expected effects and side effects have been discussed.
- Fertility preservation has been discussed.
- Informed consent has been given by patient, parents, or guardians.[10,11]

Once transgender adolescents are started on pubertal suppression, regular monitoring should occur at 3-month intervals with physical examination to include

- Height
- Weight
- Tanner staging

Laboratory testing should be ordered at baseline and then every 3 months to assess

- Hormone levels: testosterone, estradiol, LH/FSH
- Metabolic testing: calcium, phosphorus, alkaline phosphatase, 25-hydroxy vitamin D
- Imaging: bone density and bone age (at baseline and yearly)[10,19]

Long-term treatment with pubertal suppression may be required to suppress hormone levels until a gonadectomy is performed.[10] This may not be an option for many patients due to cost, and GnRH analogs typically are stopped earlier.[20]

For transgender youth who present later in adolescence (Tanner stage 4 or 5), this is past the opportunity for pubertal suppression but male transgender patients may be started on treatment with testosterone and female transgender patients may be started on antiandrogen treatment and estradiol (discussed later).[10,11,21]

Fertility Considerations

Transgender adolescents should be counseled regarding the possible loss of fertility prior to pubertal suppression or hormonal treatment.[10] GnRH analogs act to suppress pituitary hormones and, therefore, their effects on the gonad halt spermatogenesis and oocyte development. To allow for fertility, GnRH analog therapy needs to be either delayed or discontinued to allow enough development for fertility preservation.[11,22] Individuals presenting for pubertal suppression or hormone treatment should be counseled regarding fertility preservation options and referred for specialty care as indicated.[10,11] For female transgender patients, sperm cryopreservation and surgical sperm extraction are preservation options, and for male transgender patients, embryo or oocyte cryopreservation may be pursued.[23] Studies have found that although many transgender youth desire to have children, few wish to have a biological child of their own,[24] and fertility preservation is underutilized, even if youth have been counseled.[25,26]

Bone Health

One of the possible risks of pubertal suppression with GnRH analogs is decreased bone mineralization because puberty is a critical time for bone accrual.[10] Bone changes have been shown during treatment with GnRH analogs for transwomen; bone density remained stable but there was a decrease in the z score in the lumbar spine and for young transgender men there was a trend of decreased bone density in the lumbar spine.[27] Treatment with estradiol has been shown to increase bone density and z scores in transwomen, but lower than age-matched and gender-matched norms. In transmen, the bone density and z scores increased in both the lumbar spine and femoral neck, but lower than prior to treatment.[28]

HORMONAL THERAPY INITIATION

For transgender adolescents after pubertal suppression, hormonal treatment with estradiol or testosterone may be started if gender dysphoria persists. A decision should be made with the treating mental health care professional, medical practitioner, patient, and family regarding the adolescent's readiness for hormone treatment initiation. This commonly occurs at approximately age 16 when the adolescent is able to properly consent for treatment.[10,11] Gender-affirming hormones have been shown to alter the physical characteristics of the transgender adolescent to align with their gender identity. A retrospective review of transgender adolescents from the Netherlands cohort who were treated with GnRH analogs with the addition of gender-affirming hormones at 16 years of age found that during the treatment course the waist-hip ratio and the body composition changed and correlated with their affirmed gender.[29] Once the pediatric endocrinologist has confirmed that there are no medical contraindications to treatment and that treatment is indicated, the mental health care provider can confirm that the transgender adolescent meets criteria for hormonal treatment, including:

- Gender dysphoria has been persistent
- All psychological, medical, or social issues addressed
- The adolescent understands the risks and benefits of treatment.
- Expected effects and side effects have been discussed.
- Informed consent has been given by the adolescent, parents, or care takers.[10,11]

There are concerns, however, that delaying puberty to an age that is much older than cisgender peers may lead to social isolation for transgender individuals as well as concerns regarding effects on bone density.[30] An alternate approach of starting hormonal treatment earlier, at age 14, is being studied in several centers.[19,30] Once adolescents are ready to begin gender-affirming hormones, they should be started with incrementally increasing doses. Doses may be adjusted until adult doses are reached.[10] Further research is needed to fully assess the psychosocial effects of gender-affirming hormones.[31]

TRANSGENDER FEMALES

Estrogen is the primary treatment of physical feminization for female transgender patients and can be found in oral, transdermal, and intramuscular forms. Estrogen therapy should be prescribed as 17β-estradiol because ethinyl estradiol is likely associated with an increased risk of deep vein thrombosis.[32] 17β-estradiol has been noted to be effective as an agent in pubertal induction for transgender girls.[33] Oral estradiol is typically the least expensive formulation but may confer a higher risk of thromboembolic disease because it undergoes first-pass metabolism in the liver,[10] although this risk is likely low.[34] For initiation of puberty, oral estradiol is started at 0.25 mg daily, and transdermal estradiol starting dose is 6.25 μg twice weekly and also can be increased every 6 months to target adult range dosing (**Fig. 1**).[10,19] There are possible adverse effects associated with estradiol treatment, and the highest risk is for thromboembolic events (**Fig. 2**).[10] Routine monitoring should take place every 3 months with physical examination:

- Height
- Weight
- Tanner staging
- Blood pressure
- Assessment for any adverse effects

Laboratory testing should include

- Hormonal studies: estradiol, testosterone, LH/FSH, prolactin
- Metabolic studies: calcium, phosphorus, alkaline phosphatase, 25-hydroxy vitamin D, complete blood cell count, liver and renal function, fasting lipids, glucose, insulin, hemoglobin A_{1c}, electrolytes
- Imaging: bone density and bone age if puberty was previously suppressed[10,19]

TRANSGENDER MALES

For male transgender patients, testosterone is used for masculinization. Testosterone is administered in its enanthate or cypionate form as an intramuscular or subcutaneous injection, with starting doses of either 12.5 mg weekly or 25 mg every 2 weeks, and doses can be gradually adjusted every 6 months to adult testosterone doses, with 50 to 100 mg weekly or 100 to 200 mg every 2 weeks.[10,19] Testosterone esters can

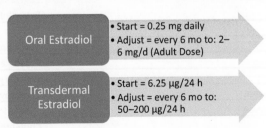

| Oral Estradiol | • Start = 0.25 mg daily
• Adjust = every 6 mo to: 2–6 mg/d (Adult Dose) |
| Transdermal Estradiol | • Start = 6.25 μg/24 h
• Adjust = every 6 mo to: 50–200 μg/24 h |

Fig. 1. Estradiol for induction of puberty.

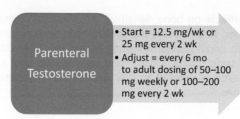

Fig. 2. Testosterone for induction of puberty.

be administered subcutaneously to reach therapeutic levels.[35] Once adult level doses are reached, a transdermal formulation of testosterone may be considered. Transdermal testosterone may be given as patch, with doses varying from 2.5 mg to 7.5 mg daily, or as a gel, with 2.5 mg to 10 mg of gel daily (see **Fig. 2**).[19] There are possible adverse effects associated with testosterone use, especially erythrocytosis (**Table 2**).[10] Similarly to female transgender patients, routine monitoring should take place every 3 months and include

- Height
- Weight
- Tanner staging
- Blood pressure
- Assessment for any adverse effects

Laboratory testing should include

- Hormonal studies: estradiol, testosterone, LH/FSH
- Metabolic studies: calcium, phosphorus, alkaline phosphatase, 25-hydroxy vitamin D, complete blood cell count, liver and renal function, fasting lipids, glucose, insulin, hemoglobin A_{1c} , electrolytes

Imaging: bone density and bone age if puberty was previously suppressed

LATE PUBERTY MANAGEMENT

Hormonal treatment of transgender youth differs for those who present later in puberty. Late puberty is considered Tanner stage 4 or 5.

For girls, breast development:

- Tanner stage 4 = areola and papilla form secondary mount
- Tanner stage 5 = nipple that projects, areola part of breast contour

Table 2 Adverse effects of cross-sex hormones	
Testosterone	**Estradiol**
Erythrocytosis	Thromboembolic disease
Liver dysfunction	Macroprolactinoma
Breast cancer	Breast cancer
Uterine cancer	Coronary artery disease
Coronary artery disease	Cerebrovascular disease
Cerebrovascular disease	Hypertriglyceridemia
Hypertension	Cholelithiasis

For boys, genital development:

- Tanner stage 4 = larger penis and glans, testes 12 mL to 15 mL, dark scrotum
- Tanner stage 5 = adult-sized penis, testes greater than 15 mL

For these individuals, there is no role for pubertal suppression, and treatment may be started with gender-affirming hormones if indicated, although GnRH agonists could be used to minimize the hormonal doses needed.[22] For male transgender patients, parenteral testosterone may be used and doses may be increased at a more rapid rate than with pubertal initiation postsuppression, starting with 75 mg intramuscular or subcutaneous every 2 weeks and increasing to 125 mg every 2 weeks after 6 months. For female transgender patients, 17β-estradiol can be prescribed with oral dosing of 1 mg daily for 6 months and it can be increased to 2 mg daily after 6 months.[10] Late pubertal female transgender patients also require the addition of antiandrogen treatment, which aids in furthering lowering of endogenous testosterone levels.[36] For this purpose in the United States, spironolactone is most commonly prescribed; it is a diuretic that is used for its antiandrogenic properties.[37] Unlike other diuretic medications, spironolactone does not cause renal potassium losses and electrolytes, including potassium, must be closely monitored during treatment.[10]

SUMMARY

Children with gender dysphoria, whose dysphoria persists and worsens with the start of puberty, can be treated with pubertal suppression with GnRH analogs. This treatment has been shown safe and effective and can allow for more time for gender exploration and unwanted physical effects of puberty. The treatment with GnRH analogs is reversible, and adolescents may proceed with either puberty of their gender assigned at birth or gender-affirming hormones with estradiol or testosterone. Further data are needed on long-term metabolic and bone outcomes for both of these groups.

REFERENCES

1. Ruble DN, Martin CL, Berenbaum SA. Gender development. In: Eisenberg N, editor. Handbook of child psychology. Social, emotional, and personality development, vol. 3. Hoboken (NJ): John Wiley & Sons; 2006. p. 858–932.
2. American Psychiatric Association. Diagnostic and statistical manual of mental disorders. 5th edition. Washington, DC: American Psychiatric Association; 2013.
3. Steensma TD, Biemond R, de Boer F, et al. Desisting and persisting gender dysphoria after childhood: a qualitative follow-up study. Clin Child Psychol Psychiatry 2011;16(4):499–516.
4. Arcelus J, Bouman WP, Van Den Noortgate W, et al. Systematic review and meta-analysis of prevalence studies in transsexualism. Eur Psychiatry 2015;30(6): 807–15.
5. Wiepjes CM, Nota NM, de Blok CJM, et al. The Amsterdam cohort of gender dysphoria study (1972-2015): trends in prevalence, treatment, and regrets. J Sex Med 2018;15(4):582–90.
6. Spack NP, Edwards-Leeper L, Feldman HA, et al. Children and adolescents with gender identity disorder referred to a pediatric medical center. Pediatrics 2012; 129(3):418–25.
7. Chen M, Fuqua J, Eugster EA. Characteristics of referrals for gender dysphoria over a 13-year period. J Adolesc Health 2016;58(3):369–71.
8. Aitken M, Steensma TD, Blanchard R, et al. Evidence for an altered sex ratio in clinic-referred adolescents with gender dysphoria. J Sex Med 2015;12(3):756–63.

9. Chiniara LN, Bonifacio HJ, Palmert MR. Characteristics of adolescents referred to a gender clinic: are youth seen now different from those in initial reports? Horm Res Paediatr 2018;89(6):434–41.
10. Hembree WC, Cohen-Kettenis PT, Gooren L, et al. Endocrine treatment of gender-dysphoric/gender-incongruent persons: an Endocrine Society* clinical practice guideline. J Clin Endocrinol Metab 2017;102(11):3869–903.
11. Coleman E, Bockting W, Botzer M, et al. Standards of care for the health of transsexual, transgender and gender-nonconforming peple version 7. Int J Transgend 2012;13:165–232.
12. Steensma TD, McGuire JK, Kreukels BP, et al. Factors associated with desistence and persistence of childhood gender dysphoria: a quantitative follow-up study. J Am Acad Child Adolesc Psychiatry 2013;52(6):582–90.
13. de Vries AL, Cohen-Kettenis PT. Clinical management of gender dysphoria in children and adolescents: the Dutch approach. J Homosex 2012;59(3):301–20.
14. Cohen-Kettenis PT, van Goozen SH. Pubertal delay as an aid in diagnosis and treatment of a transsexual adolescent. Eur Child Adolesc Psychiatry 1998;7(4):246–8.
15. de Vries AL, Steensma TD, Doreleijers TA, et al. Puberty suppression in adolescents with gender identity disorder: a prospective follow-up study. J Sex Med 2011;8(8):2276–83.
16. Lee PA. Central precocious puberty. An overview of diagnosis, treatment, and outcome. Endocrinol Metab Clin North Am 1999;28(4):901–18, xi.
17. Carel JC, Eugster EA, Rogol A, et al. Consensus statement on the use of gonadotropin-releasing hormone analogs in children. Pediatrics 2009;123(4):e752–62.
18. Schagen SE, Cohen-Kettenis PT, Delemarre-van de Waal HA, et al. Efficacy and safety of gonadotropin-releasing hormone agonist treatment to suppress puberty in gender dysphoric adolescents. J Sex Med 2016;13(7):1125–32.
19. Rosenthal SM. Approach to the patient: transgender youth: endocrine considerations. J Clin Endocrinol Metab 2014;99(12):4379–89.
20. Stevens J, Gomez-Lobo V, Pine-Twaddell E. Insurance coverage of puberty blocker therapies for transgender youth. Pediatrics 2015;136(6):1029–31.
21. Spack NP. Management of transgenderism. JAMA 2013;309(5):478–84.
22. Hembree WC, Cohen-Kettenis P, Delemarre-van de Waal HA, et al. Endocrine treatment of transsexual persons: an Endocrine Society clinical practice guideline. J Clin Endocrinol Metab 2009;94(9):3132–54.
23. De Roo C, Tilleman K, T'Sjoen G, et al. Fertility options in transgender people. Int Rev Psychiatry 2016;28(1):112–9.
24. Strang JF, Jarin J, Call D, et al. Transgender youth fertility attitudes questionnaire: measure development in nonautistic and autistic transgender youth and their parents. J Adolesc Health 2018;62(2):128–35.
25. Nahata L, Tishelman AC, Caltabellotta NM, et al. Low fertility preservation utilization among transgender youth. J Adolesc Health 2017;61(1):40–4.
26. Chen D, Simons L, Johnson EK, et al. Fertility preservation for transgender adolescents. J Adolesc Health 2017;61(1):120–3.
27. Klink D, Caris M, Heijboer A, et al. Bone mass in young adulthood following gonadotropin-releasing hormone analog treatment and cross-sex hormone treatment in adolescents with gender dysphoria. J Clin Endocrinol Metab 2015;100(2):E270–5.
28. Vlot MC, Klink DT, den Heijer M, et al. Effect of pubertal suppression and cross-sex hormone therapy on bone turnover markers and bone mineral apparent density (BMAD) in transgender adolescents. Bone 2017;95:11–9.

29. Klaver M, de Mutsert R, Wiepjes CM, et al. Early Hormonal treatment affects body composition and body shape in young transgender adolescents. J Sex Med 2018;15(2):251–60.

30. Rosenthal SM. Transgender youth: current concepts. Ann Pediatr Endocrinol Metab 2016;21(4):185–92.

31. Chew D, Anderson J, Williams K, et al. Hormonal treatment in young people with gender dysphoria: a systematic review. Pediatrics 2018;141(4) [pii:e20173742].

32. Toorians AW, Thomassen MC, Zweegman S, et al. Venous thrombosis and changes of hemostatic variables during cross-sex hormone treatment in transsexual people. J Clin Endocrinol Metab 2003;88(12):5723–9.

33. Hannema SE, Schagen SEE, Cohen-Kettenis PT, et al. Efficacy and safety of pubertal induction using 17beta-Estradiol in transgirls. J Clin Endocrinol Metab 2017;102(7):2356–63.

34. Asscheman H, T'Sjoen G, Lemaire A, et al. Venous thrombo-embolism as a complication of cross-sex hormone treatment of male-to-female transsexual subjects: a review. Andrologia 2014;46(7):791–5.

35. Spratt DI, Stewart II, Savage C, et al. Subcutaneous injection of testosterone is an effective and preferred alternative to intramuscular injection: demonstration in female-to-male transgender patients. J Clin Endocrinol Metab 2017;102(7):2349–55.

36. Prior JC, Vigna YM, Watson D. Spironolactone with physiological female steroids for presurgical therapy of male-to-female transsexualism. Arch Sex Behav 1989;18(1):49–57.

37. Corvol P, Michaud A, Menard J, et al. Antiandrogenic effect of spirolactones: mechanism of action. Endocrinology 1975;97(1):52–8.

Transfeminine Hormone Therapy

Oksana Hamidi, DO[a], Caroline J. Davidge-Pitts, MB, BCh[b],*

KEYWORDS

- Anti-androgen • Estrogen • Gender-affirming hormone therapy
- Transgender male-to-female • Gender incongruence • Gender dysphoria

KEY POINTS

- Feminizing hormone therapy (FHT) induces physical feminization, improving gender dysphoria and quality of life in transgender women.
- Prior to initiation of FHT, transgender women should be counseled on the potential adverse risks and deleterious effects on fertility.
- Long-term health monitoring for age-appropriate cancer screening, including breast and prostate; cardiovascular disease; and osteoporosis, should be continued.
- FHT is associated with increased risk of venous thromboembolism and ischemic stroke; therefore, transdermal preparations are preferred in older patients and those at high risk.

INTRODUCTION

The goal of feminizing hormone therapy (FHT) is to induce physical changes that match and affirm an individual's gender identity and to achieve and maintain normal physiologic levels of female sex hormones, thereby alleviating the distress associated with gender dysphoria/gender incongruence.[1,2] Guidelines published several organizations (World Professional Association for Transgender Health, Endocrine Society, and the University of California, San Francisco, Center of Excellence for Transgender Health) provide assistance to clinicians who care for transgender people. Previous studies have demonstrated that gender-affirming medical and surgical interventions alleviate gender dysphoria and lead to improved well-being.[3,4] Despite successful medical transition, many transgender individuals continue to experience low quality of life and remain vulnerable to mental health concerns.[5,6] Therefore, a multidisciplinary team that includes mental health providers is critical when caring for

Disclosure Statement: The authors have nothing to disclose.
[a] Division of Endocrinology and Metabolism, University of Texas Southwestern Medical Center, 2001 Inwood Road, Dallas, TX 75235, USA; [b] Division of Endocrinology, Diabetes, and Nutrition, Mayo Clinic, 200 First Street Southwest, Rochester, MN 55902, USA
* Corresponding author.
E-mail address: Davidge-Pitts.Caroline@mayo.edu

transgender individuals because collaborative efforts between appropriate health care providers optimize the chance for successful outcomes.

CRITERIA FOR INITIATION OF FEMINIZING HORMONE THERAPY

Prior to proceeding with FHT, the following criteria should be fulfilled[2]:

1. Persistent, well-documented gender dysphoria/gender incongruence
2. Capacity to make a fully informed decision and to consent to treatment
3. Age of majority if younger, follow criteria for adolescents
4. Reasonably well-controlled mental and medical health concerns, if present

BASELINE EVALUATION

Endocrine Society guidelines recommend evaluation of medical conditions that could be exacerbated by FHT. Unsupervised use of hormone therapy is strongly discouraged, and attempt at tobacco use reduction or discontinuation should occur.[2]

During the initial evaluation, the health care provider should obtain detailed personal and family medical history, paying particular attention to active or prior hormone-sensitive malignancies (eg, prostate cancer and breast cancer), history of liver dysfunction, cardiovascular disease (CVD)/stroke, and active thromboembolic disease or its risk factors. Per clinical judgment, baseline laboratory work-up should assess lipid profile, fasting glucose, complete blood cell count, liver enzymes, electrolytes, prolactin, and sex steroid hormones. The authors routinely assess immunization status (including human papillomavirus); evaluate for substance use, HIV and other sexually transmitted infections, and fertility desire; and screen for potentially harmful treatment approaches.

EXPECTED CHANGES IN RESPONSE TO FEMINIZING HORMONE THERAPY

Although precise onset and timing of feminizing physical changes in response to medical interventions are not well defined, most physical changes begin within a few months and continue to progress over a course of 2 years to 3 years (**Fig. 1**).[1,2] Expectations should be discussed with each patient prior to initiation of FHT.

Breast development is an important outcome for transgender women. A recent study of 229 transgender women, median age 28 years, revealed that most breast development occurs in the first 6 months, with mean breast-chest difference increasing from 4.1 cm ± 2.9 cm at baseline to 7.9 cm ± 3.1 cm after 1 year of FHT.[7] Approximately half of the cohort did not achieve a cup size greater than AAA, and only 3.6% of women achieved a cup size greater than A.[7] There were no predictive factors of total breast development, including age, weight change, smoking, body mass index, serum estradiol levels, and route of estrogen administration. Limitations of the study include primarily Caucasian cohort and the use of cyproterone acetate, which is not prescribed in the United States. Up to 60% of transgender women describe low satisfaction with breast development and seek breast augmentation surgery.[8] Although progestins are requested to augment breast development, to date there are no data to support their role in breast development outcomes.[9]

TREATMENT REGIMENS

The approach to FHT is not uniform and depends on the health care system, differences in the regional availability of estrogens and antiandrogens, and cost

Breast development
Onset: 3–6 mo
Maximum effect: 2–3 y

Voice
No change

Body composition
Weight gain, fat redistribution,
↓Lean muscle mass and
strength
↑Visceral fat, ↑fat mass
Onset: 3–6 mo
Maximum effect: 1–3 y

Reproductive system
Testicular atrophy (onset: 3–6
mo), ↓prostate size,
↓sperm count and quality
Maximum effect: >3 y

Hair
↓Male pattern baldness
Onset: 1–3 mo
↓Softer facial and body hair,
↓terminal hair growth
Onset: 6–12 mo
Maximum effect: 4–5 y

Skin
Skin softening, ↓sebum and
acne
Onset: 3–6 mo

Sexual health
↓Libido and spontaneous
erections
Onset: 1–3 mo
Maximum effect: 3–6 mo

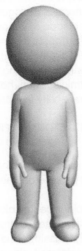

Fig. 1. Feminizing effects in transgender women.

considerations (**Table 1**).[10] A typical regimen includes therapy to lower and/or block testosterone (antiandrogens and gonadotropin-releasing hormone [GnRH] analogs) along with estrogen to inhibit testosterone secretion and provide feminizing effects.

ESTROGEN THERAPY (ROUTE/DOSE/MONITORING)

Estrogen lowers testosterone secretion from the testes by inhibiting the hypothalamic pituitary gonadal axis. Estrogen also induces feminizing physical changes. **Table 1** reviews estrogen preparations and doses. There are no robust data comparing safety and efficacy of estrogen options in transgender women. 17β-Estradiol, the most

Table 1 Gender-affirming hormone therapy in transgender women		
	Route	Dose
Estradiol	Oral	2.0–6.0 mg daily
Estradiol valerate Estradiol cypionate	Intramuscular	2–20 mg intramuscularly every 1–2 wk
Estradiol patch	Transdermal	0.025–0.2 mg/d
Estradiol gel	Transdermal (0.06% or 0.1%)	0.75 mg daily
Spironolactone	Oral	100–300 mg daily in divided doses
Cyproterone acetate	Oral	25–50 mg daily
Leuprolide Histrelin Goserelin	Subcutaneous injection or implant	3.75 mg subcutaneously monthly or 11.25 mg subcutaneously every 3 mo

Data from Hembree WC, Cohen-Kettenis PT, Gooren L, et al. Endocrine treatment of gender-dysphoric/gender-incongruent persons: an endocrine society clinical practice guideline. J Clin Endocrinol Metab 2017;102(11):3887.

commonly prescribed estrogen, is theoretically associated with smaller risk of thromboembolism than synthetic estrogens and can be measured and monitored with commercial estradiol assays. In postmenopausal cisgender women, oral estrogen was associated with higher risk of a first episode of venous thromboembolism (VTE) (relative risk [RR] = 1.63), deep vein thrombosis (RR = 2.09), and stroke (RR = 1.24) compared with transdermal estrogen.[11] Transdermal, sublingual, and parenteral preparations are believed less thrombogenic by avoiding the first-pass effect, as opposed to oral estrogens. These routes of administration, however, are associated with more rapid absorption, peaks, and wider variability in estradiol concentrations.[12]

ANTIANDROGEN THERAPY (SPIRONOLACTONE, CYPROTERONE ACETATE, FINASTERIDE, AND BICALUTAMIDE)

Antiandrogens block androgen action and also can have an inhibitory effect on testosterone secretion. Spironolactone and cyproterone acetate are the most common antiandrogens used in FHT.

Spironolactone is a mineralocorticoid receptor blocker, which has antagonistic effects on the androgen receptor at higher doses. Spironolactone also inhibits the secretion of testosterone from the testes, possibly due to progestin and estrogen-like effects.[13] It is generally safe and well tolerated, although it can induce hyperkalemia.

Cyproterone acetate is a progestin with androgen-blocking properties. Adverse effects include hepatotoxicity, depression, and multifocal meningiomas.[14,15] Although cyproterone acetate is widely used in Europe, it is not available in the United States.

5α-Reductase inhibitors (eg, finasteride) block conversion of testosterone to dihydrotestosterone, a potent androgen.[16] 5α-Reductase inhibitors have been associated with adverse mood alterations, therefore are not recommended as a first-line agent. Androgen receptor antagonists (eg, bicalutamide) do not reduce testosterone levels and are not recommended as a first-line therapy because of potentially serious hepatotoxic effects.[17]

GONADOTROPIN-RELEASING HORMONE ANALOGS (EG, LEUPROLIDE, GOSERELIN, AND HISTRELIN)

GnRH analogs reduce the secretion of luteinizing hormone and follicle-stimulating hormone, which in turn decreases stimulation of testicular testosterone production. When combined with estrogen, GnRH analogs effectively lower testosterone levels with few side effects.[18] GnRH analogs can be considered in transgender individuals who cannot tolerate antiandrogens or in patients who require a lower dose of estrogen, such as older patients and those at risk of VTE or vascular disease. In practice, the use of GnRH analogs is limited in many countries because of their prohibitive cost.

PROGESTINS

The role of progestins in FHT remains unclear, although it is often requested to enhance breast development and improve mood. To date, only a few low-quality studies have attempted to address the role of progestin in breast development among transgender women, with no definitive conclusion.[9] Currently, progestins are not recommended as part of standard FHT by Endocrine Society guidelines.

MONITORING

FHT is associated with few adverse events; however, it should be prescribed and monitored by an experienced medical provider.[19] On initiation of FHT, sex steroid hormones should be maintained in the normal physiologic range for cisgender women: estradiol, 100 pg/mL to 200 pg/mL (and not exceeding 400 pg/mL), and testosterone less than 50 ng/dL. Sex steroid hormone levels should be monitored every 3 months during the first year of FHT and then once or twice yearly thereafter.[2]

Physical changes induced by FHT should be reviewed at the initial visit and each subsequent follow-up. Health care providers should monitor weight and blood pressure; perform physical examinations; and assess tobacco use, symptoms of depression, and side effects (**Table 2**). In transgender women taking spironolactone, serum potassium should be monitored every 3 months to 4 months in the first 2 years and then annually.[2]

For those who undergo gonadectomy, testosterone levels decline and antiandrogens can be discontinued. Serum testosterone can be measured within a month after surgery to confirm that the concentrations are low (<50 pg/mL) and that testosterone-lowering medications no longer are indicated. The dose of estradiol should be maintained at a level that also is adequate to prevent osteoporosis, hot flashes, and mood disorders.[20]

EFFECTS OF ESTROGEN/ANTIANDROGEN ON TESTICULAR FUNCTION AND FERTILITY

Many transgender individuals desire biological children and seek fertility preservation.[21] Therefore, all transgender women should be informed about fertility effects of hormone treatment and counseled regarding options for fertility preservation prior to initiating hormone therapy.[1,2]

FERTILITY PRESERVATION

In transgender women who initiate FHT after puberty, prolonged estrogen and antiandrogen treatment results in reduction of the testicular volume and reduced production and quality of sperm. Current fertility preservation options for transgender women include sperm cryopreservation, surgical sperm extraction, and testicular tissue cryopreservation (experimental).[22] If fertility preservation is not feasible and low-quality semen samples are used, assisted reproduction techniques, such as in vitro

Table 2		
Monitoring of transgender women on feminizing hormone therapy		
Monitoring	**Frequency**	**Goal**
Monitor for feminizing signs and symptoms and development of side effects	Every 3 mo in the first year and then 1 to 2 times per year	Development of feminizing physical changes with no side effects
Measure testosterone and estradiol concentrations	Every 3 mo	Serum testosterone concentration: <50 ng/dL Serum estradiol concentration: 100–200 pg/mL
Serum electrolytes (if using spironolactone)	Every 3 mo in the first year and then yearly	Potassium within normal reference range Stable renal function

Data from Hembree WC, Cohen-Kettenis PT, Gooren L, et al. Endocrine treatment of gender-dysphoric/gender-incongruent persons: an endocrine society clinical practice guideline. J Clin Endocrinol Metab 2017;102(11):3890.

fertilization and intracytoplasmic sperm injection, are needed.[23] Health care providers caring for transgender women should counsel their patients that FHT is not an effective method of contraception.

VENOUS THROMBOEMBOLISM

The lifetime risk of venous thrombosis in transgender women has been reported to range between 1% and 5%.[24] Many studies evaluated small cohorts over short follow-up periods, however. Data from early studies in transgender women in the Netherlands, with a mean 10-year follow-up, suggest that the lifetime thromboembolic event prevalence was approximately 5%.[25] In a small study of 50 transgender women, thromboembolic events were reported in 3 (6%) patients.[26] In another retrospective study of 165 transgender women, the prevalence of thromboembolism was 1.2%, with higher frequency attributed to the use of conjugated estrogens compared with other estrogen preparations.[8] Subsequently published data indicate that the risk of thromboembolic disease is much lower and that the cause of the increased risk of thromboembolic disease in the earlier cohort was largely related to the use of ethinyl estradiol.[27] Several other reports from European centers have suggested that the lifetime risk of thromboembolism is very low, approximately 1%.[18,28,29] Nevertheless, in a recent large electronic medical record–based study of more than 2000 transgender women (mostly on oral estradiol), the incidence rate for VTE was higher than both cisgender male and cisgender female control groups, and the difference was more pronounced with increased follow up, with 2-year and 8-year risk differences of 4.1 (95% CI, 1.6–6.7) and 16.7 (CI, 6.4–27.5) per 1000 persons relative to cisgender men and 3.4 (CI, 1.1–5.6) and 13.7 (CI, 4.1–22.7) per 1000 persons relative to cisgender women.[30]

The risk of VTE associated with FHT can be mitigated by electing alternative routes of hormone administration. For instance, current use of oral estrogens increased risk for thromboembolism in cisgender women by 2-fold to 3-fold, whereas the risk remained unchanged among women using transdermal estradiol.[31] In another study, there was a 50% reduction in risk of VTE after switching all transgender women older than 40 years from oral to transdermal estradiol.[25] Additionally, no cases of thromboembolism were reported in 162 transgender women treated with transdermal estrogen and 5 years of follow-up, further supporting the concept that transdermal preparations pose lower thrombogenic risks as opposed to oral estrogens.[25] Transgender individuals seeking FHT should be informed about the potential risk of thromboembolic disease due to estrogen treatment and advised on modifiable factors, such as abstaining from tobacco use, maintaining lean body weight, and controlling hypertension. Individuals with a history of VTE or thrombophilia may require addition of an anticoagulant to mitigate risk of ongoing estradiol therapy.

DYSLIPIDEMIA

A meta-analysis summarizing the effects of sex steroids on lipid profile in transgender women (3231 transgender female participants in 23 studies) showed no statistically significant difference in serum low-density lipoprotein (LDL) cholesterol, high-density lipoprotein (HDL) cholesterol and total cholesterol over a course of gender-affirming hormone therapy, whereas serum triglycerides were significantly higher at greater than or equal to 24 months of treatment (31.9 mg/dL; 95% CI, 3.9–59.9 mg/dL).[32] In a subgroup analysis comparing transgender women treated with oral estrogens versus transdermal estrogens, the group on oral estrogens experienced an increase of 28.2 mg/dL (95% CI, 0.5–55.9 mg/dL) versus a decrease of 4.8 mg/dL (95% CI, −21.2–11.6 mg/dL) in the transdermal group (P = .04) at 3 months to

6 months of follow-up.[32] All other lipid profile parameters, including HDL cholesterol and LDL cholesterol, remained unchanged. Whether these statistically significant changes in triglycerides pose important clinical implications remains debatable.

DIABETES

Transgender women may be at increased risk of developing type 2 diabetes mellitus, although there are no outcome studies looking at the development of diabetes as an endpoint. An increased prevalence of type 2 diabetes mellitus was noted among transgender women on gender-affirming hormone therapy compared with age-matched cisgender men and cisgender women.[33] FHT may lead to an increase in markers of insulin resistance.[34]

HYPERTENSION

The effects of FHT on systolic blood pressure and diastolic blood pressure are inconsistent. Although most studies show an increase in systolic blood pressure in response to estrogen therapy, these findings have not been observed by others.[34–37] Diastolic blood pressure may increase or remain unchanged.[34–37] For instance, in a multicenter 1-year prospective study in 53 transgender women, systolic blood pressure decreased from 125.1 mm Hg ± 13.8 mm Hg to 118.8 mm Hg ± 13.9 mm Hg (P = .005) in 40 transgender women on oral estrogen and from 131.6 mm Hg ± 15.8 mm Hg to 128.8 mm Hg ± 15.5 mm Hg (P = .47) in 13 transgender women on transdermal estrogens.[35] In another study in 150 transgender women, systolic blood pressure (from 115.5 mm Hg to 121.9 mm Hg) and diastolic blood pressure (from 72.9 mm Hg to 76.6 mm Hg) significantly increased but remained within normal range at 24 months of oral estradiol or transdermal estradiol with cyproterone acetate treatment.[36] Similar increases in systolic blood pressure and diastolic blood pressure measurements were observed by others.[34,37]

LIVER

Although earlier studies reported liver enzyme elevations in up to 15% of transgender women receiving FHT,[38,39] subsequent data concluded that liver derangements were largely related to alcohol misuse and viral hepatitis rather than therapy itself.[25] Although estrogen therapy seems safe with respect to its effects on the liver, periodic monitoring of liver enzymes is advisable.[2]

MORTALITY

Current FHT regimens are effective and carry a low risk for side effects and adverse events at short-term follow-up. Transgender women, however, may have a higher rate of cardiovascular mortality compared with cisgender women.[3,40] In a short-term multicenter 1-year prospective study in 53 transwomen on oral estradiol or transdermal estradiol and cyproterone acetate, no deaths or severe adverse events were observed.[35] In a long-term cohort study of 966 transgender women on FHT (oral estradiol or transdermal estradiol and cyproterone acetate) followed for a median of 18.5 years, overall mortality was 51% higher than in the general cisgender women, primarily attributed to increased mortality rates due to suicide, AIDS, CVD, and drug abuse.[40] Use of ethinyl estradiol was associated with an independent threefold increased risk of cardiovascular death.[40] In a recent report, mortality rate in transgender men and transgender women was approximately 9.3% over a 10-year follow-up period, with CVD and cancer as the first and second leading causes of death, respectively.[41]

PROSTATE CANCER SCREENING

The incidence of prostate cancer in transgender women with medically induced and/ or surgically induced hypogonadism is rare, with only a few reported cases.[42–45] A single case of prostate cancer was identified in a large population of 2306 transgender women receiving with gender-affirming hormone therapy over 2 decades of follow-up period (mean follow-up of 21.4 years).[46] Yet, transgender women remain susceptible to malignancies of natal reproductive organs. The reported incidence is likely underestimated because patients and their health care providers might not realize that the prostate is not removed during gender-affirming surgery. Additionally, it remains unclear whether estrogens and antiandrogens are protective against development of prostate cancer. Lastly, incidence of prostate cancer might be affected by the age of initiation of FHT and duration of follow-up, because 1 of the reported patients developed metastatic disease 31 years after starting hormone treatment.[42] Moreover, when diagnosed in this population, prostate cancer seems to behave aggressively, complicated by the fact that PSA measurement may not be reliable in those who are receiving FHT.[42,46] Therefore, screening for prostate cancer with regular PSA testing and rectal examinations should be advisable in transgender women beginning at age 50 years, until long-term large cohort data are available for evidence-based recommendations.

BREAST CANCER

The association between the development of breast cancer and estrogen in cisgender women is complex and is contingent on the dose, duration, age at exposure, and other modifiable and nonmodifiable risk factors, such as excess weight, alcohol use, family history, and genetics. The incidence of breast cancer increases with age and with duration of exposure to sex hormones in cisgender women.

Breast cancer occurs in transgender women who develop breast tissue in response to gender-affirming hormone treatment. The estimated rate of breast cancer among transgender women is 4.1 per 100,000 person-years (95% CI, 0.8–13.0), lower than expected in cisgender women (170.0 per 100,000 person-years) but similar to cisgender men (1.2 per 100,000 patient-years).[47] In a large cohort of 5135 transgender female veterans, there was no increased risk of breast cancer compared with the general population.[48] In another study of 2571 transgender women on FHT, there were 25 cases of breast cancer, with the increased breast cancer risk compared with cisgender men but similar to cisgender women.[49] Several studies have shown that the cases of breast cancer observed in transgender women occurred at a younger age and after relatively short duration of estrogen exposure.[50,51] Due to paucity of data in transgender women, however, there is no clear evidence-based guideline on when screening for breast cancer with mammography should commence. Screening for breast cancer in transgender women could begin at the same age as recommended for cisgender women, in particular those who have been on FHT for 5 years to 10 years, and should be available to those who desire screening.[52] Screening should begin earlier in those with additional risk factors, such as a family history of breast cancer, BRCA2 mutation, Klinefelter syndrome, and others.

OSTEOPOROSIS AND BONE HEALTH

Estrogen is a key regulator of bone metabolism, and estradiol concentrations directly predict fractures in cisgender men and cisgender women.[53] Among transgender women treated with estrogens and antiandrogens, who undergo gonadectomy, estrogen treatment has been shown to counter bone loss mediated by testosterone deprivation.[54] Although there are no data on prevalence of fragility fractures among transgender women, prior to gender-affirming hormone therapy, transgender women have lower bone density, lower muscle mass and strength, and lean body mass compared with control cisgender men.[55] Moreover, up to 16% of transgender women have T scores below −2.5 at the hip and/or spine prior to initiation of gender-affirming hormone therapy.[56] The cause of low bone density in transgender women is poorly understood, with potential correlating factors including poor nutrition, vitamin D deficiency, and limited physical activity.[56] Estrogen hormone therapy in transgender women has been shown to increase bone mineral density at the femoral neck, radius, lumbar spine, and total body, indicating that skeletal status is preserved during gender-affirming hormone therapy, despite substantial muscle loss.[55] A meta-analysis and systematic review of 392 transgender women showed that there was a statistically significant increase in lumbar spine bone density at 12 months and 24 months after initiation of FHT.[57] Despite lack of established guidelines on the timing of bone mineral testing, an initial screening dual-energy x-ray absorptiometry may be checked after age 40 years if risk factors are present or if there is a personal history of fracture.[58]

ESTROGEN AND PROLACTIN

Estrogen therapy can stimulate the growth of pituitary lactotrophs. Several reports described development of prolactinoma after long-term high-dose estrogen therapy, with hyperprolactinemia and pituitary enlargement affecting up to 20% to 30% of the subjects.[59–61] Follow-up studies demonstrated that although hyperprolactinemia developed in transgender women on estrogen and antiandrogen (cyproterone acetate), baseline and postgonadectomy prolactin levels were compatible and no hyperprolactinemia was identified after gonadectomy.[59] Thus, in transgender women, prolactin increased during presurgical FHT but normalized after gonadectomy, which indicates that hyperprolactinemia was likely induced by cyproterone acetate, and not by estrogen. Similar concerns about hyperprolactinemia associated with cyproterone acetate, which has not been reported with spironolactone, have been reported by other investigators.[62,63]

Current Endocrine Society guidelines suggest periodic monitoring of prolactin levels in transgender women treated with estrogens. Although a few case studies reported on prolactinomas with FHT, similar concerns were not reported in large cohorts of estrogen-treated persons. Therefore, the risk of developing prolactinoma is likely low. Yet, because signs and symptoms of prolactinoma may be masked in transgender women on gender-affirming hormone therapy, those with persistently increasing prolactin levels despite stable or reduced estrogen may need radiologic examination of the pituitary gland. Transgender individuals who also receive psychotropic medications may have increased prolactin levels.[59]

CARE FOR POSTMENOPAUSAL-AGE TRANSGENDER WOMEN (INCLUDING CARDIOVASCULAR DISEASE AND ISCHEMIC STROKE)

The use of estrogen (0.625 mg/d of conjugated equine estrogen) and medroxyprogesterone in otherwise healthy postmenopausal cisgender women increases the risk of ischemic stroke, breast cancer, and coronary heart disease.[64–66] The use of estrogen without medroxyprogesterone does not affect the incidence of coronary heart disease and possibly reduced breast cancer risk.[67] In postmenopausal cisgender women, older age at initiation of hormone replacement therapy (age >65 years), longer duration of hormone therapy (>5 years), and higher dose of estrogen therapy were associated with greater risk of stroke and VTE.[68]

To date, evidence on the risks of FHT in transgender women greater than 50 years of age is lacking. Ideal data would come from randomized controlled trials in the same population; however, placebo control is not ethical in transgender individuals. Outcome data are limited by hormone regimens, type, and route, and cardiovascular risk profiles are difficult to match. The goal of FHT in aging transgender women is to promote feminizing hormone effects and limit venous thrombosis, cardiovascular, and breast cancer risks. Continuing full-dose estradiol in menopausal age transgender women may pose risks. Therefore, it is important to discuss the possibility of gradual taper of estradiol dose and/or switching from oral to safer transdermal/parenteral estradiol without leading to increased masculinization in individuals without gonadectomy.

CARDIOVASCULAR DISEASE

FHT has potential CVD risk in transgender women.[69] Data on CVD outcomes in transgender women on FHT are limited. Male gender assigned at birth is an independent predictor of CVD, but it remains uncertain how FHT has an impact on the CVD outcomes in transgender women, especially in those with preexisting atherosclerosis.[70] In transgender women, myocardial infarction rates were higher than in cisgender women, but similar to cisgender men, with incidence rates of 2.9 in transgender women versus 1.8 in age-matched cisgender women and 0.9 in age-matched cisgender men.[30] Risk of myocardial infarction is particularly high in transgender women who have additional risk factors, such as metabolic disease, tobacco use, or taking oral ethinyl estradiol.[30]

ISCHEMIC STROKE

Data on the effects of FHT on the incidence of stroke are limited. In aging postmenopausal cisgender women, hormone therapy is associated with increased risk of stroke. In the Women's Health Initiative study, hazard ratios for stroke were 1.37 for the conjugated equine estrogens and medroxyprogesterone arm and 1.35 for conjugated equine estrogens alone, or 9 to 11 strokes per 10,000 person-years.[17] In postmenopausal cisgender women who began hormone therapy more than 10 years after menopause, RR of stroke was 1.21, whereas no adverse effect was noted in whose who initiated hormone therapy less than 10 years after menopause or in postmenopausal women with preexisting CVD.[71] Risk of stroke with hormone therapy in postmenopausal cisgender women depends on the dose and route of estrogen delivery.[68,72]

In transgender women, risk of ischemic stroke accumulates with the exposure to FHT. Risk of ischemic stroke is higher with use of oral estrogens as opposed to transdermal preparations. In a systematic review, 8 cases of stroke were reported in a pooled population of 859 individuals on estrogen therapy.[32] The recent transfeminine cohort study showed that incidence rate of ischemic stroke was 4.8 as opposed to 1.2 in reference men and 1.9 in reference women, with a particular increase in incidence after 6 years of treatment.[30]

MANAGEMENT OF FEMINIZING HORMONE THERAPY PRIOR TO SURGERY

In most individuals, estradiol can be continued prior to surgeries that do not result in significant immobility. For higher-risk surgeries, or for patients who are high risk for VTE, discontinuation of estrogen therapy for 2 weeks to 6 weeks prior to surgery may be needed. If estrogen discontinuation is not acceptable, the route of estrogen administration could be switched to transdermal in higher-risk patients. Postoperatively, patients should be treated with prophylaxis for deep vein thrombosis and should not reinitiate estrogen until fully ambulatory. Meanwhile, urgent surgery requires thrombosis prophylaxis with low-molecular-weight heparin.[10] To further reduce the risk for thrombogenesis and other postsurgical complications, transgender women should be counseled about modifiable risk factors prior to surgery, such as body weight, smoking, and drug misuse.[58] Of significant importance, overweight or obese patients are at increased likelihood of poor perioperative outcomes after common outpatient plastic surgical procedures.[73] Thus, engaging the patients early in the course of their gender-affirming transition is of crucial importance.

HIV TREATMENT AND FEMINIZING HORMONE THERAPY

Transgender women as a group are at the highest risk for HIV infections, with the incidence of HIV in this population 3.4 to 7.8 per 100 person-years.[74–76] There is a concern about potential interactions between antiretroviral regimens and FHT. A recent analysis revealed that transgender women receiving emtricitabine and tenofovir for preexposure prophylaxis were less likely to have detectable drug levels compared with cisgender men.[77] In light of these potential interactions, HIV-positive transgender women receiving feminizing hormones may need tailored antiretroviral regimen.

SUMMARY

FHT remains a foundation in care for transgender women. Available guidelines provide assistance in the initial assessment, prescribing, and monitoring of FHT. Overall, FHT is safe and effective in inducing physical feminization. High-quality studies are needed to further expand current knowledge of long-term outcomes of FHT.

REFERENCES

1. Coleman E, Bockting W, Botzer M, et al. Standards of care for the health of transsexual, transgender, and gender-nonconforming people, version 7. Int J Transgend 2012;13(4):165–232.
2. Hembree WC, Cohen-Kettenis PT, Gooren L, et al. Endocrine treatment of gender-dysphoric/gender-incongruent persons: an endocrine society clinical practice guideline. J Clin Endocrinol Metab 2017;102(11):3869–903.
3. Dhejne C, Lichtenstein P, Boman M, et al. Long-term follow-up of transsexual persons undergoing sex reassignment surgery: cohort study in Sweden. PLoS One 2011;6(2):e16885.
4. Murad MH, Elamin MB, Garcia MZ, et al. Hormonal therapy and sex reassignment: a systematic review and meta-analysis of quality of life and psychosocial outcomes. Clin Endocrinol 2010;72(2):214–31.
5. Nobili A, Glazebrook C, Arcelus J. Quality of life of treatment-seeking transgender adults: a systematic review and meta-analysis. Rev Endocr Metab Disord 2018; 19(3):199–220.
6. Jellestad L, Jäggi T, Corbisiero S, et al. Quality of life in transitioned trans persons: a retrospective cross-sectional cohort study. Biomed Res Int 2018;2018: 8684625.
7. de Blok CJM, Klaver M, Wiepjes CM, et al. Breast development in transwomen after 1 year of cross-sex hormone therapy: results of a prospective multicenter study. J Clin Endocrinol Metab 2017;103(2):532–8.

8. Seal L, Franklin S, Richards C, et al. Predictive markers for mammoplasty and a comparison of side effect profiles in transwomen taking various hormonal regimens. J Clin Endocrinol Metab 2012;97(12):4422–8.

9. Wierckx K, Gooren L, T'sjoen G. Clinical review: Breast development in trans women receiving cross-sex hormones. J Sex Med 2014;11(5):1240–7.

10. Wylie K, Knudson G, Khan SI, et al. Serving transgender people: clinical care considerations and service delivery models in transgender health. Lancet 2016;388(10042):401–11.

11. Mohammed K, Abu Dabrh AM, Benkhadra K, et al. Oral vs transdermal estrogen therapy and vascular events: a systematic review and meta-analysis. J Clin Endocrinol Metab 2015;100(11):4012–20.

12. Price TM, Blauer KL, Hansen M, et al. Single-dose pharmacokinetics of sublingual versus oral administration of micronized 17β-estradiol. Obstet Gynecol 1997;89(3):340–5.

13. Deedwania PC, Mather PJ. Drug & device selection in heart failure. New Delhi (India): JP Medical Ltd; 2014.

14. Gil M, Oliva B, Timoner J, et al. Risk of meningioma among users of high doses of cyproterone acetate as compared with the general population: evidence from a population-based cohort study. Br J Clin Pharmacol 2011;72(6):965–8.

15. Gazzeri R, Galarza M, Gazzeri G. Growth of a meningioma in a transsexual patient after estrogen–progestin therapy. N Engl J Med 2007;357(23):2411–2.

16. Spack NP. Management of transgenderism. JAMA 2013;309(5):478–84.

17. Manson JE, Chlebowski RT, Stefanick ML, et al. Menopausal hormone therapy and health outcomes during the intervention and extended poststopping phases of the Women's Health Initiative randomized trials. JAMA 2013;310(13):1353–68.

18. Dittrich R, Binder H, Cupisti S, et al. Endocrine treatment of male-to-female transsexuals using gonadotropin-releasing hormone agonist. Exp Clin Endocrinol Diabetes 2005;113(10):586–92.

19. Weinand JD, Safer JD. Hormone therapy in transgender adults is safe with provider supervision; A review of hormone therapy sequelae for transgender individuals. J Clin Transl Endocrinol 2015;2(2):55–60.

20. Gooren L, Lips P. Conjectures concerning cross-sex hormone treatment of aging transsexual persons. J Sex Med 2014;11(8):2012–9.

21. T'Sjoen G, Van Caenegem E, Wierckx K. Transgenderism and reproduction. Curr Opin Endocrinol Diabetes Obes 2013;20(6):575–9.

22. De Roo C, Tilleman K, T'Sjoen G, et al. Fertility options in transgender people. Int Rev Psychiatry 2016;28(1):112–9.

23. Ettner R, Monstrey S, Coleman E. Principles of transgender medicine and surgery. New York: Routledge; 2016.

24. Shatzel JJ, Connelly KJ, DeLoughery TG. Thrombotic issues in transgender medicine: a review. Am J Hematol 2017;92(2):204–8.

25. Van Kesteren PJ, Asscheman H, Megens JA, et al. Mortality and morbidity in transsexual subjects treated with cross-sex hormones. Clin Endocrinol (Oxf) 1997;47(3):337–43.

26. Wierckx K, Mueller S, Weyers S, et al. Long-term evaluation of cross-sex hormone treatment in transsexual persons. J Sex Med 2012;9(10):2641–51.

27. Gooren LJ, Giltay EJ, Bunck MC. Long-term treatment of transsexuals with cross-sex hormones: extensive personal experience. J Clin Endocrinol Metab 2008;93(1):19–25.

28. Ott J, Kaufmann U, Bentz E-K, et al. Incidence of thrombophilia and venous thrombosis in transsexuals under cross-sex hormone therapy. Fertil Steril 2010; 93(4):1267–72.
29. Deutsch MB, Bhakri V, Kubicek K. Effects of cross-sex hormone treatment on transgender women and men. Obstet Gynecol 2015;125(3):605.
30. Getahun D, Nash R, Flanders WD, et al. Cross-sex hormones and acute cardiovascular events in transgender persons: a cohort study. Ann Intern Med 2018; 169(4):205–13.
31. Canonico M, Plu-Bureau G, Lowe GD, et al. Hormone replacement therapy and risk of venous thromboembolism in postmenopausal women: systematic review and meta-analysis. BMJ 2008;336(7655):1227–31.
32. Maraka S, Singh Ospina N, Rodriguez-Gutierrez R, et al. Sex steroids and cardiovascular outcomes in transgender individuals: a systematic review and meta-analysis. J Clin Endocrinol Metab 2017;102(11):3914–23.
33. Wierckx K, Elaut E, Declercq E, et al. Prevalence of cardiovascular disease and cancer during cross-sex hormone therapy in a large cohort of trans persons: a case–control study. Eur J Endocrinol 2013;169(4):471–8.
34. Elbers JM, Giltay EJ, Teerlink T, et al. Effects of sex steroids on components of the insulin resistance syndrome in transsexual subjects. Clin Endocrinol (Oxf) 2003; 58(5):562–71.
35. Wierckx K, Van Caenegem E, Schreiner T, et al. Cross-sex hormone therapy in trans persons is safe and effective at short-time follow-up: results from the E uropean N etwork for the I nvestigation of G ender I ncongruence. J Sex Med 2014; 11(8):1999–2011.
36. Quirós C, Patrascioiu I, Mora M, et al. Effect of cross-sex hormone treatment on cardiovascular risk factors in transsexual individuals. Experience in a specialized unit in Catalonia. Endocrinol Nutr 2015;62(5):210–6.
37. Colizzi M, Costa R, Scaramuzzi F, et al. Concomitant psychiatric problems and hormonal treatment induced metabolic syndrome in gender dysphoria individuals: a 2 year follow-up study. J Psychosomatic Res 2015;78(4):399–406.
38. Asscheman H, Gooren L, Eklund P. Mortality and morbidity in transsexual patients with cross-gender hormone treatment. Metabolism 1989;38(9):869–73.
39. Meyer WJ, Webb A, Stuart CA, et al. Physical and hormonal evaluation of transsexual patients: a longitudinal study. Arch Sex Behav 1986;15(2):121–38.
40. Asscheman H, Giltay EJ, Megens JA, et al. A long-term follow-up study of mortality in transsexuals receiving treatment with cross-sex hormones. Eur J Endocrinol 2011;164(4):635–42.
41. Blosnich JR, Brown GR, Wojcio S, et al. Mortality among veterans with transgender-related diagnoses in the veterans health administration, FY2000–2009. LGBT Health 2014;1(4):269–76.
42. Turo R, Jallad S, Prescott S, et al. Metastatic prostate cancer in transsexual diagnosed after three decades of estrogen therapy. Can Urol Assoc J 2013;7(7–8): E544.
43. Haarst V. Metastatic prostatic carcinoma in a male-to-female transsexual. Br J Urol 1998;81(5):776.
44. Dorff TB, Shazer RL, Nepomuceno EM, et al. Successful treatment of metastatic androgen-independent prostate carcinoma in a transsexual patient. Clin Genitourin Cancer 2007;5(5):344–6.
45. Thurston AV. Carcinoma of the prostate in a transsexual. Br J Urol 1994;73(2):217.

46. Gooren L, Morgentaler A. Prostate cancer incidence in orchidectomised male-to-female transsexual persons treated with oestrogens. Andrologia 2014;46(10): 1156–60.

47. Gooren LJ, T'Sjoen G. Endocrine treatment of aging transgender people. Rev Endocr Metab Disord 2018;19(3):253–62.

48. Brown GR, Jones KT. Incidence of breast cancer in a cohort of 5,135 transgender veterans. Breast Cancer Res Treat 2015;149(1):191–8.

49. de Blok Christel J, Wiepjes CM, Nota NM, et al. Breast cancer in transgender persons receiving gender affirming hormone treatment: results of a nationwide cohort study. Paper presented at: 20th European Congress of Endocrinology. Barcelona, Spain, May 19, 2018.

50. Gooren L, Bowers M, Lips P, et al. Five new cases of breast cancer in transsexual persons. Andrologia 2015;47(10):1202–5.

51. Gooren LJ, van Trotsenburg MA, Giltay EJ, et al. Breast cancer development in transsexual subjects receiving cross-sex hormone treatment. J Sex Med 2013; 10(12):3129–34.

52. Maglione KD, Margolies L, Jaffer S, et al. Breast cancer in male-to-female transsexuals: use of breast imaging for detection. AJR Am J Roentgenol 2014;203(6): W735–40.

53. Cauley JA. Estrogen and bone health in men and women. Steroids 2015;99:11–5.

54. Van Kesteren P, Lips P, Gooren LJ, et al. Long-term follow-up of bone mineral density and bone metabolism in transsexuals treated with cross-sex hormones. Clin Endocrinol 1998;48(3):347–54.

55. Van Caenegem E, Wierckx K, Taes Y, et al. Preservation of volumetric bone density and geometry in trans women during cross-sex hormonal therapy: a prospective observational study. Osteoporos Int 2015;26(1):35–47.

56. Van Caenegem E, Taes Y, Wierckx K, et al. Low bone mass is prevalent in male-to-female transsexual persons before the start of cross-sex hormonal therapy and gonadectomy. Bone 2013;54(1):92–7.

57. Singh-Ospina N, Maraka S, Rodriguez-Gutierrez R, et al. Effect of sex steroids on the bone health of transgender individuals: a systematic review and meta-analysis. J Clin Endocrinol Metab 2017;102(11):3904–13.

58. Tangpricha V, den Heijer M. Oestrogen and anti-androgen therapy for transgender women. Lancet Diabetes Endocrinol 2017;5(4):291–300.

59. Nota N, Dekker M, Klaver M, et al. Prolactin levels during short-and long-term cross-sex hormone treatment: an observational study in transgender persons. Andrologia 2017;49(6):e12666.

60. Kovacs K, Stefaneanu L, Ezzat S, et al. Prolactin-producing pituitary adenoma in a male-to-female transsexual patient with protracted estrogen administration. A morphologic study. Arch Pathol Lab Med 1994;118(5):562–5.

61. Cunha F, Domenice S, Câmara V, et al. Diagnosis of prolactinoma in two male-to-female transsexual subjects following high-dose cross-sex hormone therapy. Andrologia 2015;47(6):680–4.

62. Defreyne J, Nota N, Pereira C, et al. Transient elevated serum prolactin in trans women is caused by cyproterone acetate treatment. LGBT Health 2017;4(5): 328–36.

63. Fung R, Hellstern-Layefsky M, Tastenhoye C, et al. Differential effects of cyproterone acetate vs spironolactone on serum high-density lipoprotein and prolactin concentrations in the hormonal treatment of transgender women. J Sex Med 2016;13(11):1765–72.

64. Manson JE, Hsia J, Johnson KC, et al. Estrogen plus progestin and the risk of coronary heart disease. N Engl J Med 2003;349(6):523–34.
65. Chlebowski RT, Hendrix SL, Langer RD, et al. Influence of estrogen plus progestin on breast cancer and mammography in healthy postmenopausal women: the Women's Health Initiative Randomized Trial. JAMA 2003;289(24):3243–53.
66. Wassertheil-Smoller S, Hendrix S, Limacher M, et al. Effect of estrogen plus progestin on stroke in postmenopausal women: the Women's Health Initiative: a randomized trial. JAMA 2003;289(20):2673–84.
67. Patterson L. Effects of conjugated equine estrogen in postmenopausal women with hysterectomy. BMJ Sex Reprod Health 2004;30(4):279.
68. Renoux C, Dell'Aniello S, Garbe E, et al. Transdermal and oral hormone replacement therapy and the risk of stroke: a nested case-control study. BMJ 2010;340: c2519.
69. Streed CG Jr, Harfouch O, Marvel F, et al. Cardiovascular disease among transgender adults receiving hormone therapy: a narrative review. Ann Intern Med 2017;167(4):256–67.
70. Goff DC, Lloyd-Jones DM, Bennett G, et al. 2013 ACC/AHA guideline on the assessment of cardiovascular risk: a report of the American College of Cardiology/American Heart Association Task Force on Practice Guidelines. J Am Coll Cardiol 2014;63(25 Part B):2935–59.
71. Boardman H, Hartley L, Eisinga A, et al. Hormone therapy for preventing cardiovascular disease in post-menopausal women. Cochrane Database Syst Rev 2015;(3):CD002229.
72. Canonico M, Carcaillon L, Plu-Bureau G, et al. Postmenopausal hormone therapy and risk of stroke: impact of the route of estrogen administration and type of progestogen. Stroke 2016;47(7):1734–41.
73. Sieffert MR, Fox JP, Abbott LE, et al. Obesity is associated with increased health care charges in patients undergoing outpatient plastic surgery. Plast Reconstr Surg 2015;135(5):1396–404.
74. Simon PA, Reback CJ, Bemis CC. HIV prevalence and incidence among male-to-female transsexuals receiving HIV prevention services in Los Angeles County. AIDS 2000;14(18):2953–5.
75. Kellogg TA, Clements-Nolle K, Dilley J, et al. Incidence of human immunodeficiency virus among male-to-female transgendered persons in San Francisco. J Acquir Immune Defic Syndr 2001;28(4):380–4.
76. Radix A, Sevelius J, Deutsch MB. Transgender women, hormonal therapy and HIV treatment: a comprehensive review of the literature and recommendations for best practices. J Int AIDS Soc 2016;19(3S2):20810.
77. Davidson A, Franicevich J, Freeman M, et al. Tom Waddell Health Center protocols for hormonal reassignment of gender 2013. Retrieved from the Tom Waddell Health Center. Available at: https://www.sfdph.org/dph/comupg/oservices/medSvs/hlthCtrs/TransGendprotocols122006.pdf. Accessed October 16, 2018.

Transmasculine Hormone Therapy

Justine Defreyne, MD[a],*, Guy T'Sjoen, MD, PhD[b]

KEYWORDS

- Testosterone • Gender-affirming hormones • Transgender men • Safety • Follow-up

KEY POINTS

- Gender-affirming hormone treatment not only leads to physical changes, it also helps to reduce mental health problems in transgender people.
- Studies evaluating short-term and middle-term results in transgender men (TM) have concluded that testosterone treatment is safe regarding cardiovascular and oncological disease, although the long-term risk has not been assessed.
- TM who do not wish to undergo surgery are advised to seek breast and cervical cancer screening according to the protocols for cisgender women.

INTRODUCTION

Population-based estimates of the number of transgender persons range from 0.5% to 1.3% for birth-assigned male persons and from 0.4% to 1.2% for birth-assigned female persons.[1] (See Michael Goodman and colleagues' article, "Size and Distribution of Transgender and Gender Non-conforming Populations: A Narrative Review," in this issue.) Currently, the number of transgender persons seeking gender-affirming care is still increasing,[2] although access to all health care services remains precarious.[3] This may lead to a higher number of transgender people postponing health care when needed (United States: 28%–56% compared with 20% of the general population), especially transgender people who had previously outed themselves as being transgender and were taking gender-affirming hormones and/or had undergone chest reconstructive surgery.[4,5] From the study by Cruz,[4] conducted in the United States in 2014, it is known that a higher number of transgender men (TM) postponed health care compared with transgender women (TW) (odds ratio 0.484).

Transgender care is still not a (strong) part of the medical curriculum,[4] which may lead to miscommunication, misinformation, not referring trans persons to the appropriate care providers, postponing health care when needed, uncontrolled hormone

The authors have nothing to disclose.
[a] Department of Endocrinology, Ghent University Hospital, Corneel Heymanslaan 10, Ghent 9000, Belgium; [b] Department of Endocrinology, Center for Sexology and Gender, Ghent University Hospital, Corneel Heymanslaan 10, Ghent 9000, Belgium
* Corresponding author.
E-mail address: justine.defreyne@ugent.be

Endocrinol Metab Clin N Am 48 (2019) 357–375
https://doi.org/10.1016/j.ecl.2019.01.004
0889-8529/19/© 2019 Elsevier Inc. All rights reserved.

use, and even self-performed gender-affirming surgery.[6] Gender-affirming hormone therapy (HT) has been proven safe and effective in transgender persons in short-term and middle-term follow-up,[7–11] with an overall improved quality of life and a decrease in psychiatric morbidities and suicide rates after initiation of gender-affirming HT.[10–17] Therefore, it is important for health care workers in both specialty and primary care to get acquainted with the medical needs of transgender persons and to understand the impact on morbidity and mortality.

INITIAL EVALUATION: CONFIRMING THE DIAGNOSIS

The Endocrine Society's "Endocrine Treatment of Gender-Dysphoric/Gender-Incongruent Persons: An Endocrine Society Clinical Practice Guideline"[18] recommends that a mental health professional or qualified health professional confirm the diagnosis of gender incongruence or gender dysphoria before the initiation of gender-affirming hormones. Timing of gender-affirming HT is discussed in collaboration with the transgender person and their health care providers. Usually, the mental health professional will ask the person to sign or give oral informed consent regarding the risks and benefits of HT. Ideally, fertility preservation options should be discussed with the transgender person before referral to the endocrinologist in order provide a sufficient time frame for decision-making and fertility preservation, if desired. The presence of mental health concerns does not necessarily exclude patients from gender-affirming hormones, although it is advised that they be reasonably well-controlled.[18] In case of contraindications for HT due to health concerns, the health care provider should provide access to nonhormonal interventions for gender dysphoria or delay therapy until the health concerns are addressed.

Gender-affirming hormonal treatment (and surgery) has been shown to reduce and, in some cases, even resolve gender dysphoria and mental health problems.[10,11,13] In addition, gender-affirming treatment increases self-reported quality of life.[17] Satisfaction rates among transgender persons are high and gender-affirming treatment is very rarely regretted.[16,17,19,20] Ideally, gender-affirming hormonal therapy is only available by prescription. However, one must realize that there is a black market for steroids, including testosterone analogues. In addition, in non-Western countries or areas where gender-affirming care is less easily available, gender-affirming HT is often self-administered without supervision by a medical professional.

Guidelines, including the World Professional Association for Transgender Health (WPATH) "Standards of Care," edition 7,[21] and the Endocrine Society guideline, advise the hormone-providing professional to screen transgender people for conditions that can be aggravated by HT before initiating gender-affirming care. Medical history should be assessed thoroughly, including history of thromboembolic diseases (eg, deep vein thrombosis, pulmonary embolism), arterial hypertension, polycythemia, and sleep apnea.[18] To maintain virilization and avoid hypogonadism symptoms (eg, osteoporosis or vasomotor symptoms), testosterone therapy is usually continued lifelong after oophorectomy, unless medical contraindications arise.

The physician who prescribes the hormones is responsible for discussing the expected effects of testosterone therapy and the possible adverse health effects, including the possible reduction in fertility (which should ideally be discussed before the patient is referred to the endocrinology department). The physician should also provide ongoing medical monitoring with regular physical and laboratory examination, and communicate as needed with the patient's primary care provider, mental health professional, surgeon, and/or other health care professionals involved.[18,21]

Because testosterone therapy may lead to reduced fertility, options for preserving fertility and/or fulfilling (a possible future) parental desire should be discussed again with the endocrinologist, before initiating gender-affirming hormones. If fertility preservation is desired, the timing should be discussed. Although it is possible for TM to preserve oocytes after the initiation of testosterone therapy, temporarily stopping testosterone administration will be required. Armuand and colleagues[22] described that most TM who temporarily interrupted testosterone to proceed with fertility preservation felt irritable or unstable and less comfortable with their bodies. Participants who regained bleeding described this feature as among the toughest parts. Therefore, it is important to discuss fertility preservation options with the mental health professional early on in the transition process, so that transgender people do not feel rushed to make decisions they may regret in the future.

GENDER-AFFIRMING HORMONES
Testosterone

TM seeking gender-affirming HT expect to change their physical appearance to better match their gender identity and expression. Desired effects can range from an androgynous presentation to maximum virilization.[18] Ideally, the gender-affirming HT is tailored to the patient's goals, the risk-to-benefit ratio of the treatment, and cooccurring morbidities, while taking into account possible social and economic issues.[21] Testosterone therapy is contraindicated in case of (desired) pregnancy or lactation. If patients are screened adequately and follow-up visits are provided regularly, testosterone therapy is safe on the short term and middle term, with very low rates of adverse events.[7,8,23–27] The hormone-prescribing physician is responsible for discussing the desired effects of testosterone therapy and possible impact on physical and mental health.

Hormonal therapy in TM consists of testosterone agents, preferably administered intramuscularly, subcutaneously, or transdermally. Testosterone regimens in TM follow the general principle of hormone replacement therapy for male hypogonadism, aiming at cisgender male reference ranges for serum testosterone levels.[18] If desired, treatment regimens can be adapted to meet transgender people's expectations. Injectable testosterone esters are the most commonly prescribed testosterone agents in TM, used in dosages of 200 to 250 mg intramuscularly or subcutaneously every 2 to 3 weeks, or lower doses weekly.[18,28,29] Another frequently used agent is long-acting testosterone undecanoate 1000 mg intramuscularly every 10 to 12 weeks.[30] Other options include topical androgen gel 1% (25–100 mg/d) or transdermal patches (2.5–10 mg/d).[18] Rarely used options for gender-affirming HT in TM include oral testosterone (testosterone undecanoate 160–240 mg/d), axillary solutions, patches, nasal sprays, buccal tablets, or pellets. Preferred options for gender-affirming HT in TM are also described in "Endocrine Treatment of Gender-Dysphoric/Gender-Incongruent Persons: An Endocrine Society Clinical Practice Guideline."[18]

As long as the therapy is supervised by a physician and patients adhere to the prescribed dose, different testosterone formulations are comparable regarding short-term safety, compliance, metabolic parameters, body composition, and general life satisfaction.[31] In the United States, long-acting testosterone undecanoate therapy can only be initiated after Risk Evaluation and Mitigation Strategy (REMS) training for both patient and provider, due to the potential risk of pulmonary oil embolism. The dose of testosterone may be increased if trough serum total testosterone levels do not reach cisgender male levels after 6 months of testosterone therapy (by increasing the injected dose or by decreasing the injection interval), with subsequent monitoring of serum hematocrit levels. The dose may be decreased if serum hematocrit levels increase above male reference ranges or if desired by the patient.

Progestational Agents

Menstrual bleeding is often experienced as uncomfortable by TM,[22,32] and can even be associated with increased feelings of anger and embarrassment.[33] Enquiring about the persistence of menstrual bleeding and the degree of inconvenience this causes should be part of the assessment. Medication to induce amenorrhea should be discussed with every transgender man early in the transition process. Suppression of menstrual bleedings is less likely in TM treated with transdermal or oral testosterone.[23] A progestational agent or a gonadotropin-releasing hormone (GnRH) analogue can be added to the treatment regimen if suppression of the menses is desired or menstrual bleeding does not cease. The most commonly used agents include oral lynestrenol 5 to 10 mg daily or medroxyprogesterone 5 to 10 mg daily. GnRH analogues are rarely used in adults because of the cost of the therapy. Other rarely used options include the use of an intrauterine device or endometrial ablation.[7] Progestational therapy can be stopped after hystero-oophorectomy.

The use of progestational agents is contraindicated in case of pregnancy, less than 6 weeks postpartum if breastfeeding, (history of) breast cancer or any gynecological cancer, unexplained vaginal bleeding, (multiple risk factors for) arterial cardiovascular disease, current or previous ischemic heart disease or stroke, acute deep venous thrombosis or pulmonary embolism, liver insufficiency, severe bile or liver diseases (including liver tumors), epilepsy with aura, and systemic lupus erythematosus (with positive or unknown antiphospholipid antibodies or severe thrombopenia), as well as use of antiretroviral ritonavir-boosted protease inhibitors, rifampicin, rifabutin, or medications to treat seizures or tuberculosis. Possible side effects include gastrointestinal discomfort, water and salt retention, weight gain, decreased sexual desire, and spotting.[34]

DESIRABLE EFFECTS

Testosterone therapy gradually induces virilization. It causes the voice to break,[35] facial and body hair appear in a male pattern,[36] the musculature becomes bulkier and more pronounced,[37] the clitoris enlarges (mean 3.83 ± 0.42 cm after 2 years of testosterone therapy),[11] and sometimes amenorrhea occurs (**Fig. 1**). Owing to these effects, most TM are being perceived by others as a cisgender man in daily life, which leads to decreasing feelings of body uneasiness.[11,13] It is important to discuss the possibilities and limitations of testosterone therapy before and during gender-affirming HT; height and bone structure will not change after puberty and testosterone therapy will not affect subcutaneous fat mass, unless physical activity is initiated or increased.[38]

Voice

Testosterone therapy leads to hypertrophy of muscle cells with a reduction of surrounding fat cells. These effects are also exerted at the level of the larynx, which results in acoustic changes.[39] Testosterone therapy in concentrations of greater than or equal to 150 µg/dL has a virilizing effect on the voice of birth-assigned women. Repeated exposure to concentrations greater than 200 µg/dL results in irreversible changes, occurring predominantly during the first 3 months of testosterone therapy.[35] Although TM are more likely to experience problems with pitch quality (incidence 10%), their voice frequently cannot be distinguished from cisgender men.[40,41] TM in whom the voice is perceived as male, report overall higher wellbeing compared with those with less gender-congruent voices.[42]

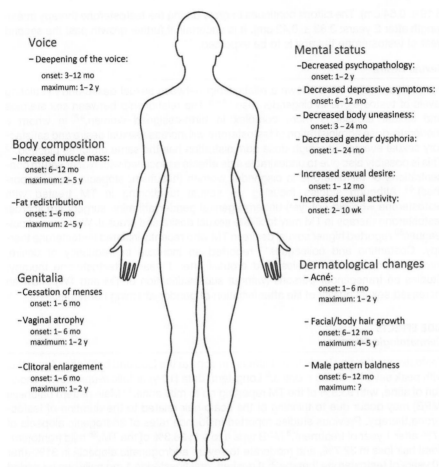

Voice
– Deepening of the voice:
    onset: 3–12 mo
    maximum: 1–2 y

Body composition
–Increased muscle mass:
    onset: 6–12 mo
    maximum: 2–5 y

–Fat redistribution
    onset: 1–6 mo
    maximum: 2–5 y

Genitalia
–Cessation of menses
    onset: 1–6 mo

–Vaginal atrophy
    onset: 1–6 mo
    maximum: 1–2 y

–Clitoral enlargement
    onset: 1–6 mo
    maximum: 1–2 y

Mental status
–Decreased psychopathology:
    onset: 1–2 y
– Decreased depressive symptoms:
    onset: 6–12 mo
– Decreased body uneasiness:
    onset: 3–24 mo
– Decreased gender dysphoria:
    onset: 1–24 mo

– Increased sexual desire:
    onset: 1–12 mo
– Increased sexual activity:
    onset: 2–10 wk

Dermatological changes
– Acné:
    onset: 1–6 mo
    maximum: 1–2 y

– Facial/body hair growth
    onset: 6–12 mo
    maximum: 4–5 y

– Male pattern baldness
    onset: 6–12 mo
    maximum: ?

Fig. 1. Virilizing effects of testosterone therapy in TM, based on observations by Wierckx and colleagues,[8] Fisher and colleagues,[11] Slabbekoorn and colleagues,[135] Toorians and colleagues,[136] and Asscheman and colleagues.[137] (*Adapted from* Hembree WC, Cohen-Kettenis PT, Gooren L, et al. Endocrine treatment of gender-dysphoric/gender-incongruent persons: an Endocrine Society clinical practice guideline. J Clin Endocrinol Metab 2017;102(11):3869–903; with permission.)

Dermatologic Effects

The pilosebaceous unit of the skin expresses both androgen and estrogen receptors, which allows testosterone to exert effects on the skin and hair of TM. Testosterone therapy leads to a desirable increase in body and facial hair. The increase is already apparent during the first year of treatment, although Ferriman-Gallwey scores are still lower during the first year of testosterone therapy compared with cisgender men.[36] Long-term data show further increasing body and facial hair growth after the first year (from median score 0.5 at baseline to 12 after 1 year and 24 after 10 years).[43]

Genitalia

Testosterone therapy increases clitoral length, which already becomes apparent after only 3 months of testosterone therapy (>60%, mean clitoral length after 3 months:

3.19 ± 0.54 cm). The clitoris continues to grow during the testosterone therapy (mean length after 2 years: 3.83 ± 0.42 cm). It is uncertain if further growth past the second year of testosterone therapy is to be expected.[11]

Sexual Desire

Numerous studies have shown a relationship between sexual desire and circulating levels of testosterone in cisgender men.[44–46] The relationship between sex steroids and sexual arousal is more complex in birth-assigned women,[47] in whom a moderate-dose administration of testosterone will increase sexual desire and satisfactory sexual events but a high-dose administration has the same effect as placebo.[48] This is possibly also due to undesirable side effects associated with higher serum concentrations of testosterone in cisgender women (hirsutism, alopecia, acne, seborrhea).[49] Although studies focusing on sexual functioning in TM treated with testosterone who did not (yet) undergo genital gender-affirming surgery are scarce, testosterone therapy in TM may facilitate sexual desire and arousal. Wierckx and colleagues[50] reported higher sexual desire in TM who recently initiated testosterone therapy. Costantino and colleagues[46] reported an increase in frequency of desire, masturbation, sexual fantasies, and arousal after 1 year of testosterone therapy. Studies on transgender persons (without substratification of TM and TW) show an increased sexual quality of life after initiation of gender-affirming hormones.[51]

SIDE EFFECTS
Dermatologic Effects

Testosterone therapy leads to an increase in acne at the face and back after 4 months, with peak severity after 6 months.[8] Long-term data (10-year follow-up) shows resolution of acne, with 93.9% of the TM reporting no to mild acne.[43] Male pattern baldness (MPB) may occur due to thinning of the scalp hair related to the duration of testosterone therapy. Previous studies reported incidence rates of androgenic alopecia of 17% after 1 year of treatment,[8] MPB type II to V in 38.3% of the TM,[36] mild frontotemporal hair loss in 32.7%, and moderate to severe androgenetic alopecia in 31% after 10 years of testosterone therapy.[52] If desired, oral finasteride 1 mg daily can be added to the treatment regimen to prevent hair loss.[53]

Genitalia

Long-term testosterone use causes vaginal and cervical atrophy, with decreased vaginal lubrication, which can result in vaginal dryness or itching and painful penetration.[54] If necessary, simple over-the-counter lubricants can be prescribed to patients reporting vaginal dryness.[55]

Cardiovascular Safety

Testosterone therapy in TM alters independent cardiac risk factors, including the lipid profile (decrease in high-density lipoprotein [HDL] cholesterol and increase in triglycerides and low-density lipoprotein [LDL] cholesterol)[8,31,56–69] and increasing serum hematocrit levels (to cisgender male reference values).[70] To date, there is scarce evidence that these changes in risk factors will result in adverse cardiovascular outcomes in TM taking testosterone therapy over short and medium (10 years) follow-up time, although data on older TM are lacking.[70–75] However, a systematic review of the literature concluded that the level of evidence was too low to allow an interpretation of the risk of testosterone therapy on morbidity (stroke, myocardial infarction, venous thromboembolism) and mortality in TM.[76] The Endocrine Society guideline[18] suggests monitoring weight, blood pressure, and lipids at regular intervals and managing cardiovascular risk factors according to population-based guidelines.

Arterial blood pressure
The available research on the impact of HT on systolic or arterial blood pressure shows conflicting results in cross-sectional and prospective studies. Emi and colleagues[77] reported higher systolic, mean arterial, and diastolic blood pressure in TM on HT, compared with TM not on testosterone. One prospective study[56] observed an increase in systolic and diastolic blood pressure in adolescent TM after 2 years of HT. Two prospective studies[59,78] reported no change in systolic over diastolic blood pressure in adult TM after initiation of HT.

Dyslipidemia
Results regarding the impact of testosterone therapy on lipid levels are often conflicting. Cross-sectional studies report higher total cholesterol levels and lower HDL levels in TM on HT compared with those without HT,[77] higher triglyceride levels in TM on HT compared with women diagnosed with polycystic ovary syndrome (PCOS)[66] and TM without HT,[66,77] and lower triglyceride levels in TM compared with TW (nonage matched).[73]

Whereas Wierckx and colleagues[8] observed an increase in total cholesterol levels over 1 year follow-up in TM on testosterone undecanoate, Jacobeit and colleagues[30,64] observed a decrease in total cholesterol levels after 12 to 18 months of testosterone undecanoate therapy. Vita and colleagues[78] observed no change in total HDL and LDL cholesterol and triglycerides over 30 months of follow-up. Whereas some studies report no change in HDL levels in TM,[30,78] others reported a decrease in HDL levels in TM.[8,56,57,62–69] Regarding LDL, 1 study observed an increase after 1 year of testosterone undecanoate therapy,[8] whereas 2 other studies[30,64] observed a decrease after 12 to 18 months of testosterone undecanoate.

It is possible that HDL metabolism is more predictive of atherogenicity, rather than circulating HDL levels.[79] Elements pointing toward increased atherogenicity in TM (increased triglyceride levels, decreased HDL2 and HDL3 levels), as well as elements pointing toward decreased atherogenicity (smaller LDL size with lower free cholesterol and phospholipid concentration, increased hepatic lipase activity and ApoC-II levels, reduced ApoA-I), have been reported.[61,69]

Metabolic syndrome
Most the studies on TM[8,31,56,67,74,80] reported no changes in insulin resistance in TM, although 2 studies[78,80] reported a decrease in fasting glucose levels after 3 to 30 months of testosterone therapy in TM. However, 1 study[8] reported a decrease in fasting insulin in TM after 1 year of testosterone therapy. Berra and colleagues[81] observed a decrease in adiponectin levels in TM 6 months after the initiation of HT. On the other hand, 1 prospective study reported an increased incidence of metabolic syndrome after 1 and 2 years of HT.[82] In addition, hyperinsulinemic-euglycemic clamp studies (a measure for peripheral insulin resistance) in TM after 4 months of HT showed a decrease in glucose utilization.[83] Elbers and colleagues[61] reported no change in fasting insulin levels or insulin sensitivity after 12 months of testosterone administration in the physiologic range in TM, although administration of supraphysiological levels of testosterone resulted in a reduced glucose uptake during a clamp test.

Markers of increased thrombotic risk
Testosterone therapy is associated with an increase in serum hemoglobin (>4.9%–12.5% range) and hematocrit (>4.4%–17.6% range) levels during the first year of

treatment, with the most pronounced increase during the first 3 months (>2.7% hematocrit, 95% CI 1.94–3.29). Serum hematocrit levels remain stable after the first year of testosterone therapy.[30,43,71] Because serum hematocrit levels can be found in the reference range of the perceived gender from 3 months after the initiation of gender-affirming hormonal treatment, it is advised to consult the reference range for men in TM after the initiation of testosterone treatment.[70] Although, theoretically, testosterone therapy increases the risk for erythrocytosis, clinically significant erythrocytosis is rare.[8,70,71] In a large prospective study by the European Network for the Investigation of Gender Incongruence (ENIGI), which included 192 TM, the maximum measured hematocrit level was 54.0% and none of the TM experienced a thromboembolic event during follow-up. There are no reasons to assume that the observed mild increase in serum hematocrit levels is associated with an increased thrombotic risk on the short term.[70] TM on testosterone undecanoate exhibit lower erythrocytosis rates compared with TM on testosterone esters or gel. Changing the treatment to testosterone undecanoate seems a valid option if the hormone-prescribing physician and/or the patient are concerned about elevated serum hematocrit levels. This may prevent unnecessary interruptions in hormonal treatment.[70] The Endocrine Society guideline[18] suggests measuring hematocrit or hemoglobin at baseline, every 3 months for the first year, and then 1 to 2 times a year.

Hepatologic Safety

According to the Endocrine Society guideline,[18] hepatotoxicity is not anticipated in TM taking parenteral or transdermal testosterone. Theoretically, an increase in liver enzymes can be observed during testosterone therapy,[18] although mainly observed in TM taking oral 17-alkylated testosterone, which is no longer recommended.[84,85] Two prospective studies reported no significant increase in liver enzymes in TM during gender-affirming HT.[30,63] During 1 year of follow-up, Wierckx and colleagues[8] described liver enzyme values exceeding twice the upper limit according to female reference ranges in 1.9% but none exceeding twice the upper limit according to male reference ranges.[8]

Bone Health

Bone mineral density (BMD) studies in transgender people have recently been meta-analyzed by Singh-Ospina and colleagues.[86] Their results report similar BMD in cisgender women and TM before testosterone therapy,[86–89] with no decrease in BMD after the initiation of testosterone therapy.[86,87,90] There was even an increase in 1 prospective study.[91] Van Caenegem and colleagues[92] described larger cortical bone size in TM after initiation of HT, compared with cisgender women. This may be due to aromatization of testosterone to estradiol and/or the androgen-mediated increase in muscle mass, thereby stimulating bone formation.[93] Van Caenegem and colleagues[92] described a positive correlation between muscle mass, strength, and trabecular and cortical parameters and bone size. The risk of osteoporotic fractures in TM has only been assessed in 1 cohort study of 53 TM (and 53 TW), reporting no fractures after 12 months of follow-up.[8] If ovariectomy has been performed, testosterone therapy is vital to preserve BMD because it prevents estrogen-deprivation related bone loss on the short term (<2 years)[31,43,87,88,90,91,94,95] and the long term (>10 years).[92,96–98] It can even result in a prospective increase in BMD at cortical sites[91] and increased cortical thickness.[99] However, in TM who underwent ovariectomy, bone loss has been described when they irregularly used or stopped androgen therapy.[89,94,96] The Endocrine Society guideline[18] suggests screening for osteoporosis in TM who stop testosterone treatment, are not compliant with HT, or who develop risks for bone loss.

Oncology

Both health care practitioners and TM themselves have expressed concern about the oncological risk of long-term testosterone therapy; however, prospective studies with sufficient sample size and follow-up duration are lacking. In the current literature, only 8 published papers assessed cancer incidence or mortality in TM. However, they reported on different populations (The Netherlands, Belgium, Sweden, and the United States) in different time periods (1989–2016).[23,25,75,100–103] No large representative multicenter prospective studies of transgender populations of sufficient duration to establish hormone-related cancer risk have been published in the current literature, although evidence suggests that transgender people are more frequently exposed to cancer risk factors, including smoking, obesity, and lack of or inadequate cancer screening (including cervical smears in TM) owing to perceived barriers for accessing health care.[104–106] Currently, the number of cancers reported in TM is relatively low compared with TW,[101,102] which may be attributable to the younger age of TM in most the published articles. As large scale epidemiologic data on long-term cancer risk in transgender people have not been published, it is advised to adhere to the screening protocols for the general population, according to birth-assigned sex if the organ is still in place.

Breast cancer

A recent systematic review[107] reported 15 cases of breast cancer in TM taking testosterone therapy.[100,107–113] Van Renterghem and colleagues[114] reported no invasive cancer in mastectomy specimens of 148 TM, although apocrine metaplasia was seen in 23.6%, lactational changes in 2%, columnar cell changes in 37.2%, sclerosing adenosis in 4.7%, fibroadenoma in 4.1%, usual ductal hyperplasia in 27%, flat epithelial atypia in 0.7%, and atypical ductal hyperplasia in 3.4%. Gooren and colleagues[100] reported a lower incidence of breast cancer in TM, compared with cisgender women (5.9 vs 155 per 100.000 person-years). The incidence of breast carcinoma after prophylactic mastectomy in cisgender women is probably less than 2%,[115] and the risk is increased in both premenopausal and postmenopausal women with higher serum testosterone levels. Aromatase can convert exogenous testosterone to estrogen in TM. However, none of the previous studies was able to find a causal relationship or association between testosterone therapy and the incidence of breast carcinoma in TM. Cases of breast cancer in TM taking testosterone occurred at ages ranging from 27 to 53 years, after 3 to 15 years of testosterone use. In epidemiologic studies in cisgender women, the association between endogenous hormones and breast cancer was stronger at older ages.[116] Routine histopathological examination of mastectomy specimens may assess whether there is an increased risk of breast carcinoma in TM compared with cisgender women.[117] To date, no large studies on breast cancer risk have been conducted in TM. The Endocrine Society[18] recommends conducting subareolar and periareolar annual breast examinations if mastectomy has been performed. If mastectomy is not performed, the American Cancer Society suggests screening by mammography, according to guidelines for birth-assigned sex. Of note, breast cancer can still occur after mastectomy has been performed and adequate screening is still recommended postmastectomy.[108,110]

Cervical cancer

The presence of human papilloma virus increases the risk for cervical cancer in birth-assigned women.[118] The relationship between serum testosterone levels and cervical cancer remains to be determined in cisgender women. One study reported a positive relationship between free testosterone and risk of invasive cervical carcinoma in pre-menopausal women, whereas cervical carcinoma was positively related to total testosterone in postmenopausal women.[119] In TM, only 3 cases of cervical cancer have been published, all in TM on testosterone therapy, although duration of administration was not always clear.[120–122] Whether testosterone therapy is associated with an increased risk for cervical cancer in TM remains unknown to date. If cervical tissue is present, the Endocrine Society guideline[18] suggests monitoring as recommended by the American College of Obstetricians and Gynecologists.[123]

Endometrial cancer

In the current literature, only 1 case of endometrial cancer has been reported in a transgender man after 7 years of testosterone therapy.[120] Grynberg and colleagues[124] retrospectively examined the genital tract histopathology of 112 TM after at least 6 months of androgen administration and reported endometrial atrophy in 45%. One sample displayed endometrial hyperplasia with a small focus of adenocarcinoma.

In postmenopausal cisgender women, an association between endometrial or ovarian cancer and higher total serum testosterone levels has been reported in observational studies.[125] This can be explained by the aromatization of testosterone into estradiol, which stimulates endometrial and ovarian epithelium proliferation, as well as by the conversion of testosterone into dihydrotestosterone (DHT) by 5α-reductase. DHT and testosterone can both increase endometrial and ovarian epidermal growth. In contrast, DHT also has antiproliferative effects on the endometrial and ovarian cancer cells, which may also lead to a decreased cancer risk.[105]

Ovarian cancer

Three cases of ovarian cancer have been reported in TM taking HT for 1 to 18 years, of which 2 cases were tested for the endometrial epidermal growth factor receptor; both were positive.[126,127] One prospective cohort study described no ovarian cancer in 112 TM after only 6 months of testosterone therapy.[124] Hage and colleagues[127] suggested stopping hormonal therapy after diagnosis of an androgen receptor–positive ovarian cancer and simultaneous salpingo-oophorectomy for any TM undergoing gender-affirming hysterectomy, whereas Dizon and colleagues[126] contradicted this by stating that there is insufficient evidence linking exogenous androgens and ovarian malignancy.

Whether testosterone therapy induces PCOS morphology of the ovarian cortex in TM remains uncertain because results are contradictory.[124,128] Ikeda and colleagues[128] described a thicker ovarian cortex, more hyperplastic collagen, ovarian stromal hyperplasia, and stromal luteinization in TM compared with control cisgender women, although the number of early-stage and antral follicles were comparable. In contrast, Grynberg and colleagues[124] reported histologic characteristics of polycystic ovaries (defined as >12 antral follicles per ovary) in 79.5% of their retrospective cohort of 112 TM after at least 6 months of HT.

In Europe, in the past, many TM included in published studies underwent hystero-oophorectomy after 12 to 18 months of HT, which reduces the cohort of TM at risk for endometrial and ovarian cancers. To establish the cancer risk in TM on testosterone therapy, large long-term cohort studies in TM who do not undergo hystero-oophorectomy, are needed.

Psychological Monitoring

Depression, suicide attempts, and anxiety rates in the transgender samples are higher compared with nontransgender samples,[129–132] although these rates decrease after initiation of gender-affirming HT[10,133] to incidence rates comparable to the general population.[10] Low social support, low self-esteem, and poorer interpersonal function are predictive factors for depression and anxiety.[131,133] Interventions offered alongside gender-affirming treatment to develop interpersonal skills also increase self-esteem, improve social support, and may reduce depression and prepare individuals for a more successful transition.[133] It is important to enquire about psychosocial well-being during each contact and to refer to a psychologist or psychiatrist if necessary. In addition, the WPATH "Standards of Care"[21] warn for a possible increased risk of destabilization of certain psychiatric disorders (including bipolar, schizoaffective, and other disorders that may include manic or psychotic symptoms) in TM with both additional risk factors and supraphysiological serum testosterone levels. The WPATH "Standards of Care" also warn for aggression or expansive mood at the beginning of an injection cycle with testosterone esters.[21] However, no increase in aggression[134] but a decrease in anxiety and depression has been observed on the initiation of gender-affirming HT in TM.[10]

SUMMARY

According to the Endocrine Society guideline,[18] follow-up should include assessment of signs of virilization and development of adverse reactions; measuring serum testosterone every 3 months until male reference ranges have reached; measuring serum hematocrit or hemoglobin at baseline, every 3 months for the first year, and then 1 to 2 times a year; and monitoring weight, blood pressure, and lipids at regular intervals. If cardiovascular risk factors emerge, they should be managed according to established population-based guidelines. BMD measurements should only be obtained when risk factors for osteoporosis exist, including stopping HT after gonadectomy. The Endocrine Society guideline[18] does not suggest monitoring liver enzymes in TM.

Studies on oncological risk in TM after the initiation of testosterone therapy remain inconclusive and lack power.[23,25,75,100–103] Therefore, is advised to adhere to the screening protocols for the general population, according to birth-assigned sex, depending on the anatomic situation.[18]

In summary, gender-affirming hormonal therapy with testosterone leads to desirable physical effects over 3 months to several years in TM, as well as reduced depression, suicide attempts, and anxiety rates[10,133] with no increased risk for aggression.[10] It is advised to discuss the options for treatment (if desired), and ask about the occurrence and need for treatment of undesirable effects. Overall, testosterone therapy in TM is considered safe on the short term and middle term, if patients adhere to the prescribed therapy and adequate endocrinological follow-up is provided.

REFERENCES

1. Winter S, Diamond M, Green J, et al. Transgender people: health at the margins of society. Lancet 2016;388:390–400.
2. Wylie K, Knudson G, Khan SI, et al. Serving transgender people: clinical care considerations and service delivery models in transgender health. Lancet 2016;388(10042):401–11.
3. Fundamental Rights Agency. Being Trans in the EU - comparative analysis of the EU LGBT survey data 2014. Luxembourg (Europe): FRA.
4. Cruz TM. Assessing access to care for transgender and gender nonconforming people: a consideration of diversity in combating discrimination. Soc Sci Med 2014;110:65–73.

5. James SE, Herman JL, Rankin S, et al. The report of the 2015 U.S. transgender survey. Washington, DC: National Center for Transgender Equality.

6. Rotondi NK, Bauer GR, Scanlon K, et al. Nonprescribed hormone use and self-performed surgeries: "do-it-yourself" transitions in transgender communities in Ontario, Canada. Am J Public Health 2013;103(10):1830–6.

7. Gorton RN, Erickson-Schroth L. Hormonal and surgical treatment options for transgender men (female-to-male). Psychiatr Clin North Am 2017;40(1):79–97.

8. Wierckx K, Van Caenegem E, Schreiner T, et al. Cross-sex hormone therapy in trans persons is safe and effective at short-time follow-up: Results from the European Network for the Investigation of Gender Incongruence. J Sex Med 2014; 11(8):1999–2011.

9. Bourgeois AL, Auriche P, Palmaro A, et al. Risk of hormonotherapy in transgender people: Literature review and data from the French Database of Pharmacovigilance. Ann Endocrinol (Paris) 2016;77(1):14–21.

10. Heylens G, Verroken C, De Cock S, et al. Effects of different steps in gender reassignment therapy on psychopathology: a prospective study of persons with a gender identity disorder. J Sex Med 2014;11(1):119–26.

11. Fisher AD, Castellini G, Ristori J, et al. Cross-sex hormone treatment and psychobiological changes in transsexual persons: two-year follow-up data. J Clin Endocrinol Metab 2016;101(11):4260–9.

12. Gorin-Lazard A, Baumstarck K, Boyer L, et al. Is Hormonal therapy associated with better quality of life in transsexuals? a cross-sectional study. J Sex Med 2012;9(2):531–41.

13. Fisher AD, Castellini G, Bandini E, et al. Cross-sex hormonal treatment and body uneasiness in individuals with gender dysphoria. J Sex Med 2014;11(3):709–19.

14. Smith YL, van Goozen SH, Cohen-Kettenis PT. Adolescents with gender identity disorder who were accepted or rejected for sex reassignment surgery: a prospective follow-up study. J Am Acad Child Adolesc Psychiatry 2001;40(4):472–81.

15. Newfield E, Hart S, Dibble S, et al. Female-to-male transgender quality of life. Qual Life Res 2006;15(9):1447–57.

16. Murad MH, Elamin MB, Garcia MZ, et al. Hormonal therapy and sex reassignment: a systematic review and meta-analysis of quality of life and psychosocial outcomes. Clin Endocrinol (Oxf) 2010;72(2):214–31.

17. Defreyne J, Motmans J, T'Sjoen G. Healthcare costs and quality of life outcomes following gender affirming surgery in trans men: a review. Expert Rev Pharmacoecon Outcomes Res 2017;17(6):543–56.

18. Hembree WC, Cohen-Kettenis PT, Gooren L, et al. Endocrine treatment of gender-dysphoric/gender-incongruent persons: an Endocrine Society clinical practice guideline. J Clin Endocrinol Metab 2017;102(11):3869–903.

19. Kuhn A, Bodmer C, Stadlmayr W, et al. Quality of life 15 years after sex reassignment surgery for transsexualism. Fertil Steril 2009;92(5).

20. Jones BA, Haycraft E, Murjan S, et al. Body dissatisfaction and disordered eating in trans people: a systematic review of the literature. Int Rev Psychiatry 2016;28(1):81–94.

21. World Professional Association for Transgender Health. WPATH standards of care. Int J Tansgend 2012;13(4):165–232.

22. Armuand G, Dhejne C, Olofsson JI, et al. Transgender men's experiences of fertility preservation: a qualitative study. Hum Reprod 2017;32(2):383–90.

23. Asscheman H, Giltay EJ, Megens JAJ, et al. A long-term follow-up study of mortality in transsexuals receiving treatment with cross-sex hormones. Eur J Endocrinol 2011;164(4):635–42.

24. Cavanaugh T, Hopwood R, Lambert C. Informed consent in the medical care of transgender and gender-nonconforming patients. AMA J Ethics 2016;18(11): 1147–55.

25. Wierckx K, Mueller S, Weyers S, et al. Long-term evaluation of cross-sex hormone treatment in transsexual persons. J Sex Med 2012;9(10):2641–51.

26. Weinand JD, Safer JD. Hormone therapy in transgender adults is safe with provider supervision; A review of hormone therapy sequelae for transgender individuals. J Clin Transl Endocrinol 2015;2(2):55–60.

27. Trum HW, Hoebeke P, Gooren LJ. Sex reassignment of transsexual people from a gynecologist's and urologist's perspective. Acta Obstet Gynecol Scand 2015; 94:563–7.

28. Olson J, Schrager SM, Clark LF, et al. Subcutaneous testosterone: an effective delivery mechanism for masculinizing young transgender men. LGBT Health 2014;1(3):165–7.

29. Spratt DI, Stewart II, Savage C, et al. Subcutaneous injection of testosterone is an effective and preferred alternative to intramuscular injection: demonstration in female-to-male transgender patients. J Clin Endocrinol Metab 2017;102(7): 2349–55.

30. Jacobeit JW, Gooren LJ, Schulte HM. Safety aspects of 36 months of administration of long-acting intramuscular testosterone undecanoate for treatment of female-to-male transgender individuals. Eur J Endocrinol 2009;161(5):795–8.

31. Pelusi C, Costantino A, Martelli V, et al. Effects of three different testosterone formulations in female-to-male transsexual persons. J Sex Med 2014;11(12): 3002–11.

32. Mitu K. Transgender reproductive choice and fertility preservation. AMA J Ethics 2016;18(11):1120.

33. Motta G, Crespi C, Mineccia V, et al. Does testosterone treatment increase anger expression in a population of transgender men? J Sex Med 2018;15(1):94–101.

34. World Health Organization, Department of Reproductive Health, World Health Organization. Medical eligibility criteria for contraceptive use. World Health Organization; 2010.

35. Bultynck C, Pas C, Defreyne J, et al. Self-perception of voice in transgender persons during cross-sex hormone therapy. Laryngoscope 2017;127(12): 2796–804.

36. Giltay EJ, Gooren LJG. Effects of sex steroid deprivation/administration on hair growth and skin sebum production in transsexual males and females. J Clin Endocrinol Metab 2000;85(8):2913–21.

37. Klaver M, de Blok C, Wiepjes C, et al. Changes in regional body fat, lean body mass and body shape in trans persons using cross-sex hormonal therapy: results from a multicenter prospective study. Eur J Endocrinol 2017;178:165–73.

38. Gooren LJ. Management of female-to-male transgender persons: medical and surgical management, life expectancy. Curr Opin Endocrinol Diabetes Obes 2014;21(3):233–8.

39. Evans S, Neave N, Wakelin D, et al. The relationship between testosterone and vocal frequencies in human males. Physiol Behav 2008;93(4–5):783–8.

40. Abitbol J, Abitbol P, Abitbol B. Sex hormones and the female voice. J Voice 1999;13(3):424–46.

41. Cosyns M, Borsel J, Wierckx K, et al. Voice in female-to-male transsexual persons after long-term androgen therapy. Laryngoscope 2014;124(6):1409–14.

42. Watt SO, Tskhay KO, Rule NO. Masculine voices predict well-being in female-to-male transgender individuals. Arch Sex Behav 2017;47:963–72.

43. Mueller A, Haeberle L, Zollver H, et al. Effects of intramuscular testosterone undecanoate on body composition and bone mineral density in female-to-male transsexuals. J Sex Med 2010;7(9):3190–8.

44. Nakamura A, Watanabe M, Sugimoto M, et al. Dose-response analysis of testosterone replacement therapy in patients with female to male gender identity disorder. Endocr J 2013;60(3):275–81.

45. Allan CA, Forbes EA, Strauss BJG, et al. Testosterone therapy increases sexual desire in ageing men with low-normal testosterone levels and symptoms of androgen deficiency. Int J Impot Res 2008;20(4):396–401.

46. Costantino A, Cerpolini S, Alvisi S, et al. A prospective study on sexual function and mood in female-to-male transsexuals during testosterone administration and after sex reassignment surgery. J Sex Marital Ther 2013;39(4):321–35.

47. Bancroft J. The endocrinology of sexual arousal. J Endocrinol 2005;186(3):411–27.

48. Davis S, Papalia M-A, Norman RJ, et al. Safety and efficacy of a testosterone metered-dose transdermal spray for treating decreased sexual satisfaction in premenopausal women: a randomized trial. Ann Intern Med 2008;148(8):569–77.

49. Somboonporn W, Davis S, Seif MW, et al. Testosterone for peri- and postmenopausal women. Cochrane Database Syst Rev 2005;(4):CD004509.

50. Wierckx K, Elaut E, Van Caenegem E, et al. Sexual desire in female-to-male transsexual persons: exploration of the role of testosterone administration. Eur J Endocrinol 2011;165(2):331–7.

51. Bartolucci C, Gómez-Gil E, Salamero M, et al. Sexual quality of life in gender-dysphoric adults before genital sex reassignment surgery. J Sex Med 2015;12(1):180–8.

52. Wierckx K, Van de Peer F, Verhaeghe E, et al. Short-and long-term clinical skin effects of testosterone treatment in trans men. J Sex Med 2014;11(1):222–9.

53. Moreno-Arrones OM, Becerra A, Vano-Galvan S. Therapeutic experience with oral finasteride for androgenetic alopecia in female-to-male transgender patients. Clin Exp Dermatol 2017;42(7):743–8.

54. Schlatterer K, Von Werder K, Stalla GK. Multistep treatment concept of transsexual patients. Exp Clin Endocrinol Diabetes 1996;104(06):413–9.

55. Leiblum S, Bachmann G, Kemmann E, et al. Vaginal atrophy in the postmenopausal woman. JAMA 1983;249(2195):1983–2198.

56. Olson-Kennedy J, Okonta V, Clark LF, et al. Physiologic response to gender-affirming hormones among transgender youth. J Adolesc Health 2017;62(4):397–401.

57. Jarin J, Pine-Twaddell E, Trotman G, et al. Cross-sex hormones and metabolic parameters in adolescents with gender dysphoria. Pediatrics 2017;139(5):e20163173.

58. Gava G, Cerpolini S, Martelli V, et al. Cyproterone acetate versus leuprolide acetate in combination with transdermal oestradiol in transwomen: a comparison of safety and effectiveness. Clin Endocrinol (Oxf) 2016;85(2):239–46.

59. Fernandez JD, Tannock LR. Metabolic effects of hormone therapy in transgender patients. Endocr Pract 2015;22(4):383–8.

60. Auer MK, Cecil A, Roepke Y, et al. 12-months metabolic changes among gender dysphoric individuals under cross-sex hormone treatment: a targeted metabolomics study. Sci Rep 2016;6:37005.

61. Elbers JMH, Giltay EJ, Teerlink T, et al. Effects of sex steroids on components of the insulin resistance syndrome in transsexual subjects. Clin Endocrinol (Oxf) 2003;58(5):562–71.

62. Elbers JMH, Asscheman H, Seidell JC, et al. Reversal of the sex difference in serum leptin levels upon cross-sex hormone administration in transsexuals. J Clin Endocrinol Metab 1997;82(10):3267–70.

63. Mueller A, Kiesewetter F, Binder H, et al. Long-term administration of testosterone undecanoate every 3 months for testosterone supplementation in female-to-male transsexuals. J Clin Endocrinol Metab 2007;92(9):3470–5.

64. Jacobeit JW, Gooren LJ, Schulte HM. Endocrinology: long-acting intramuscular testosterone undecanoate for treatment of female-to-male transgender individuals. J Sex Med 2007;4(5):1479–84.

65. McCredie RJ, McCrohon JA, Turner L, et al. Vascular reactivity is impaired in genetic females taking high-dose androgens. J Am Coll Cardiol 1998;32(5):1331–5.

66. Cupisti S, Giltay EJ, Gooren LJ, et al. The impact of testosterone administration to female-to-male transsexuals on insulin resistance and lipid parameters compared with women with polycystic ovary syndrome. Fertil Steril 2010;94(7):2647–53.

67. Chandra P, Basra SS, Chen TC, et al. Alterations in lipids and adipocyte hormones in female-to-male transsexuals. Int J Endocrinol 2010;2010 [pii:945053].

68. Deutsch MB, Bhakri V, Kubicek K. Effects of cross-sex hormone treatment on transgender women and men. Obstet Gynecol 2015;125(3):605–10.

69. Wultsch A, Kaufmann U, Ott J, et al. Profound changes in sex hormone levels during cross-sex hormone therapy of transsexuals do not alter serum cholesterol acceptor capacity. J Sex Med 2015;12(6):1436–9.

70. Defreyne J, Vantomme B, Van Caenegem E, et al. Prospective evaluation of hematocrit in gender-affirming hormone treatment: results from European Network for the Investigation of Gender Incongruence. Andrology 2018;6:446–54.

71. Velho I, Fighera TM, Ziegelmann PK, et al. Effects of testosterone therapy on BMI, blood pressure, and laboratory profile of transgender men: a systematic review. Andrology 2017;5(5):881–8.

72. Gooren LJ, Giltay EJ. Men and women, so different, so similar: observations from cross-sex hormone treatment of transsexual subjects. Andrologia 2014;46(5):570–5.

73. Gooren LJ, Wierckx K, Giltay EJ. Cardiovascular disease in transsexual persons treated with cross-sex hormones: reversal of the traditional sex difference in cardiovascular disease pattern. Eur J Endocrinol 2014;170(6):809–19.

74. Maraka S, Singh Ospina N, Rodriguez-Gutierrez R, et al. Sex steroids and cardiovascular outcomes in transgender individuals: a systematic review and meta-analysis. J Clin Endocrinol Metab 2017;102(11):3914–23.

75. Van Kesteren PJM, Asscheman H, Megens JAJ, et al. Mortality and morbidity in transsexual subjects treated with cross-sex hormones. Clin Endocrinol (Oxf) 1997;47(3):337–43.

76. Elamin MB, Garcia MZ, Murad MH, et al. Effect of sex steroid use on cardiovascular risk in transsexual individuals: A systematic review and meta-analyses. Clin Endocrinol (Oxf) 2010;72(1):1–10.

77. Emi Y, Adachi M, Sasaki A, et al. Increased arterial stiffness in female-to-male transsexuals treated with androgen. J Obstet Gynaecol Res 2008;34(5):890–7.

78. Vita R, Settineri S, Liotta M, et al. Changes in hormonal and metabolic parameters in transgender subjects on cross-sex hormone therapy: a cohort study. Maturitas 2018;107:92–6.

79. Wu FCW, von Eckardstein A. Androgens and coronary artery disease. Endocr Rev 2003;24(2):183–217.

80. Giltay EJ, Toorians AWFT, Sarabjitsingh AR, et al. Established risk factors for coronary heart disease are unrelated to androgen-induced baldness in female-to-male transsexuals. J Endocrinol 2004;180(1):107–12.

81. Berra M, Armillotta F, D'emidio L, et al. Testosterone decreases adiponectin levels in female to male transsexuals. Asian J Androl 2006;8(6):725–9.

82. Colizzi M, Costa R, Scaramuzzi F, et al. Concomitant psychiatric problems and hormonal treatment induced metabolic syndrome in gender dysphoria individuals: a 2 year follow-up study. J Psychosom Res 2015;78(4):399–406.

83. Polderman KH, Gooren LJ, Asscheman H, et al. Induction of insulin resistance by androgens and estrogens. J Clin Endocrinol Metab 1994;79(1):265–71.

84. Bird D, Vowles K, Anthony PP. Spontaneous rupture of a liver cell adenoma after long term methyltestosterone: report of a case successfully treated by emergency right hepatic lobectomy. Br J Surg 1979;66(3):212–3.

85. Westaby D, Paradinas FJ, Ogle SJ, et al. Liver damage from long-term methyltestosterone. Lancet 1977;310(8032):261–3.

86. Singh-Ospina N, Maraka S, Rodriguez-Gutierrez R, et al. Effect of sex steroids on the bone health of transgender individuals: a systematic review and meta-analysis. J Clin Endocrinol Metab 2017;102(11):3904–13.

87. Van Caenegem E, Wierckx K, Taes Y, et al. Body composition, bone turnover, and bone mass in trans men during testosterone treatment: 1-year follow-up data from a prospective case-controlled study (ENIGI). Eur J Endocrinol 2015;172(2):163–71.

88. Haraldsen IR, Haug E, Falch J, et al. Cross-sex pattern of bone mineral density in early onset gender identity disorder. Horm Behav 2007;52(3):334–43.

89. Miyajima T, Kim YT, Oda H. A study of changes in bone metabolism in cases of gender identity disorder. J Bone Miner Metab 2012;30(4):468–73.

90. Wiepjes CM, Vlot MC, Klaver M, et al. Bone mineral density increases in trans persons after 1 year of hormonal treatment: a multicenter prospective observational study. J Bone Miner Res 2017;32(6):1252–60.

91. Turner A, Chen TC, Barber TW, et al. Testosterone increases bone mineral density in female-to-male transsexuals: a case series of 15 subjects. Clin Endocrinol (Oxf) 2004;61(5):560–6.

92. Van Caenegem E, Wierckx K, Taes Y, et al. Bone mass, bone geometry, and body composition in female-to-male transsexual persons after long-term cross-sex hormonal therapy. J Clin Endocrinol Metab 2012;97(7):2503–11.

93. Frost HM. Bone's mechanostat: a 2003 update. Anat Rec 2003;275(2):1081–101.

94. Goh HHV, Ratnam SS. Effects of hormone deficiency, androgen therapy and calcium supplementation on bone mineral density in female transsexuals. Maturitas 1997;26(1):45–52.

95. Meriggiola MC, Armillotta F, Costantino A, et al. Effects of testosterone undecanoate administered alone or in combination with letrozole or dutasteride in female to male transsexuals. J Sex Med 2008;5(10):2442–53.

96. Van Kesteren P, Lips P, Gooren LJG, et al. Long-term follow-up of bone mineral density and bone metabolism in transsexuals treated with cross-sex hormones. Clin Endocrinol (Oxf) 1998;48(3):347–54.

97. Ruetsche AG, Kneubuehl R, Birkhaeuser MH, et al. Cortical and trabecular bone mineral density in transsexuals after long-term cross-sex hormonal treatment: a cross-sectional study. Osteoporos Int 2005;16(7):791–8.

98. Schlatterer K, Auer DP, Yassouridis A, et al. Transsexualism and osteoporosis. Exp Clin Endocrinol Diabetes 1998;106(05):365–8.

99. Lips P, Van Kesteren PJ, Asscheman H, et al. The effect of androgen treatment on bone metabolism in female-to-male transsexuals. J Bone Miner Res 1996; 11(11):1769–73.

100. Gooren L, Bowers M, Lips P, et al. Five new cases of breast cancer in transsexual persons. Andrologia 2015;47(10):1202–5.

101. Wierckx K, Elaut E, Declercq E, et al. Prevalence of cardiovascular disease and cancer during cross-sex hormone therapy in a large cohort of trans persons: a case-control study. Eur J Endocrinol 2013;169(4):471–8.

102. Dhejne C, Lichtenstein P, Boman M, et al. Long-term follow-up of transsexual persons undergoing sex reassignment surgery: cohort study in Sweden. PLoS One 2011;6(2):e16885.

103. Brown GR, Jones KT. Incidence of breast cancer in a cohort of 5,135 transgender veterans. Breast Cancer Res Treat 2015;149(1):191–8.

104. Fredriksen-Goldsen KI, Cook-Daniels L, Kim H-J, et al. Physical and mental health of transgender older adults: an at-risk and underserved population. Gerontologist 2013;54(3):488–500.

105. Braun H, Nash R, Tangpricha V, et al. Cancer in transgender people: evidence and methodological considerations. Epidemiol Rev 2017;39(1):93–107.

106. Peitzmeier SM, Khullar K, Reisner SL, et al. Pap test use is lower among female-to-male patients than non-transgender women. Am J Prev Med 2014;47(6): 808–12.

107. Stone JP, Hartley RL, Temple-Oberle C. Breast cancer in transgender patients: a systematic review. part 2: female to male. Eur J Surg Oncol 2018;44:1463–8.

108. Nikolic DV, Djordjevic ML, Granic M, et al. Importance of revealing a rare case of breast cancer in a female to male transsexual after bilateral mastectomy. World J Surg Oncol 2012;10(1):280.

109. Burcombe RJ, Makris A, Pittam M, et al. Breast cancer after bilateral subcutaneous mastectomy in a female-to-male trans-sexual. Breast 2003;12(4):290–3.

110. Shao T, Grossbard ML, Klein P. Breast cancer in female-to-male transsexuals: two cases with a review of physiology and management. Clin Breast Cancer 2011;11(6):417–9.

111. Brown GR. Breast cancer in transgender veterans: a ten-case series. LGBT Health 2015;2(1):77–80.

112. Katayama Y, Motoki T, Watanabe S, et al. A very rare case of breast cancer in a female-to-male transsexual. Breast Cancer 2016;23(6):939–44.

113. Gooren LJ, van Trotsenburg MAA, Giltay EJ, et al. Breast cancer development in transsexual subjects receiving cross-sex hormone treatment. J Sex Med 2013; 10(12):3129–34.

114. Van Renterghem SMJ, Van Dorpe J, Monstrey SJ, et al. Routine histopathological examination after female-to-male gender-confirming mastectomy. Br J Surg 2018;105(7):885–92.

115. Willemsen HW, Kaas R, Peterse JH, et al. Breast carcinoma in residual breast tissue after prophylactic bilateral subcutaneous mastectomy. Eur J Surg Oncol 1998;24(4):331–2.

116. Key TJ, Appleby PN, Reeves GK, et al. Circulating sex hormones and breast cancer risk factors in postmenopausal women: reanalysis of 13 studies. Br J Cancer 2011;105(5):709.

117. Van Renterghem S, Van Dorpe J, T'Sjoen G, et al. Histopathology of transgender breast specimens: expect the unexpected! Virchows Arch 2017;471:S60.

118. Gillison ML, Chaturvedi AK, Lowy DR. HPV prophylactic vaccines and the potential prevention of noncervical cancers in both men and women. Cancer 2008;113(S10):3036–46.

119. Rinaldi S, Plummer M, Biessy C, et al. Endogenous sex steroids and risk of cervical carcinoma: results from the EPIC study. Cancer Epidemiol Prev Biomarkers 2011;20:2532–40.

120. Urban RR, Teng NNH, Kapp DS. Gynecologic malignancies in female-to-male transgender patients: the need of original gender surveillance. Am J Obstet Gynecol 2011;204(5):e9–12.

121. Driák D, Samudovsky M. Could a man be affected with carcinoma of cervix?- The first case of cervical carcinoma in trans-sexual person (FtM)-case report. Acta Medica (Hradec Kralove) 2005;48(1):53.

122. Taylor ET, Bryson MK. Cancer's margins: trans* and gender nonconforming people's access to knowledge, experiences of cancer health, and decision-making. LGBT Health 2016;3(1):79–89.

123. Saslow D, Solomon D, Lawson HW, et al. American Cancer Society, American Society for Colposcopy and Cervical Pathology, and American Society for Clinical Pathology screening guidelines for the prevention and early detection of cervical cancer. CA Cancer J Clin 2012;62(3):147–72.

124. Grynberg M, Fanchin R, Dubost G, et al. Histology of genital tract and breast tissue after long-term testosterone administration in a female-to-male transsexual population. Reprod Biomed Online 2010;20(4):553–8.

125. Allen NE, Key TJ, Dossus L, et al. Endogenous sex hormones and endometrial cancer risk in women in the European Prospective Investigation into Cancer and Nutrition (EPIC). Endocr Relat Cancer 2008;15(2):485–97.

126. Dizon DS, Tejada-Berges T, Koelliker S, et al. Ovarian cancer associated with testosterone supplementation in a female-to-male transsexual patient. Gynecol Obstet Invest 2006;62(4):226–8.

127. Hage JJ, Dekker J, Karim RB, et al. Ovarian cancer in female-to-male transsexuals: report of two cases. Gynecol Oncol 2000;76(3):413–5.

128. Ikeda K, Baba T, Noguchi H, et al. Excessive androgen exposure in female-to-male transsexual persons of reproductive age induces hyperplasia of the ovarian cortex and stroma but not polycystic ovary morphology. Hum Reprod 2012;28(2):453–61.

129. Clements-Nolle K, Marx R, Katz M. Attempted suicide among transgender persons: the influence of gender-based discrimination and victimization. J Homosex 2006;51(3):53–69.

130. Bockting WO, Miner MH, Swinburne Romine RE, et al. Stigma, mental health, and resilience in an online sample of the US transgender population. Am J Public Health 2013;103(5):943–51.

131. Budge SL, Adelson JL, Howard KAS. Anxiety and depression in transgender individuals: the roles of transition status, loss, social support, and coping. J Consult Clin Psychol 2013;81(3):545.

132. Reisner SL, Poteat T, Keatley J, et al. Global health burden and needs of transgender populations: a review. Lancet 2016;388(10042):412–36.

133. Witcomb GL, Bouman WP, Claes L, et al. Levels of depression in transgender people and its predictors: results of a large matched control study with transgender people accessing clinical services. J Affect Disord 2018;235:308–15.
134. Defreyne J, T'sjoen G, Bouman WP, et al. Prospective evaluation of self-reported aggression in transgender persons. J Sex Med 2018;15(5):768–76.
135. Slabbekoorn D, Van Goozen SH, Gooren LJ, et al. Effects of cross-sex hormone treatment on emotionality in transsexuals. Int J Transgenderism 2001;5:3.
136. Toorians A, Thomassen M, Zweegman S, et al. Venous thrombosis and changes of hemostatic variables during cross-sex hormone treatment in transsexual people. J Clin Endocrinol Metab 2003;88(12):5723–9.
137. Asscheman H, Gooren LJG, Assies J, et al. Prolactin levels and pituitary enlargement in hormone-treated male-to-female transsexuals. Clin Endocrinol (Oxf) 1988;28(6):583–8.

Primary Care in Transgender Persons

Brittany L. Whitlock, BS[a], Elizabeth S. Duda, BA[a], Molly J. Elson, BA[a],
Paul Parker Schwab, BBA[a], Ogul Ersin Uner, BA[a], Shawn Wen, MS[a],
Jason S. Schneider, MD[b,*,1]

KEYWORDS

• Transgender • Primary care • Prevention • Screening

KEY POINTS

• The preventive health care needs of transgender persons are nearly identical to the rest of the population.
• Special consideration should be given to the impact of gender-affirming hormone regimens and surgical care on preventive screenings.
• To avoid creating additional barriers to access, special attention must be given to creating a welcoming and inclusive health care system for transgender persons.
• Providers must consider the unique impact that a gender identity and expression different from the assigned gender at birth affects patient-provider interactions, including the history, physical examination, and diagnostic testing.

INTRODUCTION

A majority of health issues affecting transgender and gender nonbinary people are no different from those of the remainder of the population. Highlighted in this article and in other articles in this special issue are topics in primary care that are unique to transgender populations. The authors use a broader view of the health care system, beyond the hospital or outpatient setting, to delineate aspects of transgender health care deserving of special consideration.

SETTING THE SCENE—CONSIDERATIONS FOR THE OFFICE

Multiple social determinants of health have a negative and disproportionate impact on transgender people: violence, economic hardship, unemployment, and housing

Conflicts of Interest: None.
Funding sources: B.L. Whitlock, E.S. Duda, M.J. Elson, P.P. Schwab, O.E. Uner, and S. Wen: None; J.S. Schneider: National Institutes of Health and Emory Medical Care Foundation.
[a] Emory University School of Medicine, 100 Woodruff Circle, Suite 231, Atlanta, GA 30322, USA;
[b] Division of General Medicine and Geriatrics, Department of Medicine, Emory University School of Medicine, 49 Jesse Hill Jr Drive Southeast, Atlanta, GA 30303, USA
[1] Senior author.
* Corresponding author.
E-mail address: jsschne@emory.edu

Endocrinol Metab Clin N Am 48 (2019) 377–390
https://doi.org/10.1016/j.ecl.2019.02.004
0889-8529/19/© 2019 Elsevier Inc. All rights reserved.

insecurity, among others.[1] Transgender people also experience prohibitive inequities when finally accessing quality health care. Many transgender people have been refused health care services due to their gender identity, and many more report delaying or avoiding health care due to past experiences of harassment in medical settings and lack of provider knowledge.[2,3] For these reasons, it is imperative that health care providers and their staff be well educated in best practices regarding the care for transgender individuals.

Staff Training

Transgender people often are subject to prejudice within all levels of the health care system, and thus the first step in delivery of transcompetent care is to establish a practice as a safe space from the first point of contact with transgender patients. Education of all health care and frontline staff on standards of respect toward transgender people is highly recommended, and discourse in the practice should reflect this training continuously.

The following topics have been suggested by the Gay & Lesbian Medical Association (GLMA) to include in a staff training program[4]:

1. Use of appropriate language when addressing or referring to patients and/or their significant others
2. Learning how to identify and challenge any internalized discriminatory beliefs about lesbian, gay, bisexual, transgender, queer, and other sexual or gender non-conforming people (LGBTQ+)
3. Basic familiarity with important LGBTQ+ health issues (eg, impacts of homophobia, discrimination, harassment, and violence; mental health and depression; substance abuse; safe sex; partner violence; HIV/sexually transmitted infections)
4. Indications and mechanisms for referral to LGBTQ+identified or LGBTQ+friendly providers

Additional resources concerning education on transgender awareness can be found in the GLMA 2005 *Guidelines for Care of Lesbian, Gay, Bisexual, and Transgender Patients.*[4]

Elements of Competent Care

There are several principles that should be followed by all staff and health care personnel to provide culturally sensitive care to transgender patients.

- Name and pronouns—always address patients by their stated name and personal pronouns.
- Privacy—prioritize patient privacy. Do not assume that partners, employers, or family members are informed of a patient's gender identity.
- Terminology—providers should be aware of and comfortable using basic terminology used by the transgender community. **Table 1** lists some basic terminology as it is most often used, but providers should be aware that the language used to discuss transgender identity is constantly evolving and should attempt to use the terminology that individual patients prefer.

Electronic Health Record

An often overlooked but essential aspect of providing quality care for transgender patients is making proper adaptations to the electronic health record (EHR) of a health system. Many transgender patients identify with a name or gender identity (GI) that is different from that assigned at birth. Making EHRs compliant with a patient's

Table 1
Definition of common terminology used in the transgender community

Term	Definition
Sex	Sex is assigned at birth to individuals based on external genitalia, internal genitalia, and chromosomes.
Gender identity	A person's intrinsic sense of self as the person relates to gender
Gender expression	Outward characteristics like clothing, behaviors, and appearance that express a person's sense of gender. This is separate from gender identity; a person may identify as one gender and express components of another.
Transgender person	An individual whose gender identity is different from the gender assigned at birth
Cisgender person	An individual whose gender identity is the same as that assigned at birth
Transmasculine person	A person who has a masculine-spectrum gender identity and was assigned female gender at birth
Transfeminine person	A person who has feminine-spectrum gender identity and was assigned male at birth
Gender dysphoria	Psychological distress caused by discrepancy between a person's gender identity and gender assigned at birth, often specifically regarding secondary sex characteristics
Nonbinary person[a]	An individual who identifies as neither male nor female but rather between the 2 extremes of the gender spectrum
Agender person[a]	An individual who identifies as having no gender or as being outside of the male-female spectrum.

[a] Some, but not all, nonbinary and agender people identify as transgender.

Adapted from Center of Excellence for Transgender Health, Department of Family and Community Medicine, University of California San Francisco. Guidelines for the Primary and Gender-Affirming Care of Transgender and Gender Nonbinary People; 2nd edition. Deutsch MB, ed. June 2016. Available at: www.transhealth.ucsf.edu/guidelines; with permission.

appropriate identifiers ensures improved communication and accurate health documentation for transgender patients and can prevent recurrent errors in identification that may deter patients from seeking care.[5]

The World Professional Association for Transgender Health released guidelines on EHR use in transgender patient care.[6] These recommendations are summarized:

1. Name, GI, and pronouns identified by patients should be regarded as demographic information, like ethnicity. The system should immediately and obviously notify the provider of a patient's relevant identifiers on opening of a patient's chart if they do not match the legally documented information. The legally documented name and gender identity can still appear on the EHR and continue to be used for billing and identity verification if the patient has not completed the legal process of name, gender, and/or gender transition.
2. The EHR should have a structured inventory of a patient's medical transition history and current anatomy. If possible, a master list of anatomic organs for each patient can allow for individualized history and physical examination templates. Future system updates may allow for anatomy-based reminders of any relevant screening procedures recommended by the US Preventive Services Task Force (USPSTF).
3. The system should be able to accommodate legal and medical transition in the EHR. This involves changing the gender and anatomic inventory included in the medical record with ease and continuously educating the staff (eg, reference laboratory) to use the correct names and pronouns. Key personnel in the health

system should be familiar with state-based requirements for legal name, gender, and/or gender marker changes.

SPECIAL CONSIDERATIONS IN THE HISTORY AND PHYSICAL

This section outlines specialized components that should be included in a new patient visit or complete history and physical with a transgender patient.

History

General principles of the history

The history should attempt to catalog medical and surgical interventions and health behaviors that may affect provided care. Most medical care sought by transgender patients, however, is unrelated to their gender identity, and it is unnecessary to discuss gender-related health at every visit. It also should be kept in mind that not all transgender patients desire alteration of their bodies through hormones or surgery. Providers should inquire about physical changes but not assume that they are desired or have occurred.

Special considerations of a sensitive history

- Past medical and surgical history
  - Organ inventory: perform an organ inventory to assess what organs and/or modifications the patient has. Do not assume a patient's anatomy based on the gender presentation.
  - Procedures: inquire regarding what, if any, gender-affirming procedures the patient has had. These may include
    - Transfeminine patients: breast augmentation, orchiectomy, vaginoplasty, labiaplasty, cosmetic procedures, electrolysis, and injectable silicone use
      - If the patient endorses use of injectable silicones, further investigate where the procedure was performed. Many transfeminine individuals participate in pumping parties, where industrial-grade silicone is injected without professional supervision.[7] Improper use of injectable silicones can lead to complications, including infection, migrating globules, pneumonitis, granulomas, and pulmonary embolism.[7]
    - Transmasculine patients: mastectomy, hysterectomy, oophorectomy, vaginectomy, and genital reconstruction
  - Health conditions: ask about past or current conditions that may affect hormone therapy. These include cardiovascular disease, diabetes mellitus, psychiatric illness, liver disease, renal disease, HIV, venous thromboembolism, and hormonally mediated cancers.
  - Complications: if a patient is receiving hormone therapy, ask about potential complications regarding treatment.
- Medications
  - Regimen: ask about hormones a patient is taking, if any. Include past hormonal regimens.
  - Dose and delivery: ask about dose and delivery methods of hormonal regimens. Screen for practices of needle sharing.
  - Acquisition: ask how a patient is acquiring hormones. Many patients are prescribed hormones, whereas others may acquire supplies via the Internet or other means.
  - Efficacy: assess efficacy of patient's current regimen. Assess whether a patient's expectations about hormonal efficacy are realistic.

- Family history
  - Conduct a thorough family history, specifically assessing for conditions affecting hormone therapy. This specifically includes venous thromboembolism, cardiovascular disease, and liver disease.[8]
  - Assess for reproductive cancer risk, including breast and endometrial cancers.
- Social history
  - Conduct a sensitive sexual history, recalling that sexual orientation is distinct from gender identity.
    - The sexual history should be a behavior-focused history that uses inclusive language about partners. Do not make assumptions about a partner's gender identity or the sexual behaviors engaged in.
    - Emphasize counseling about safe sex practices and sexually transmitted infection (STI) risk reduction. HIV and other sexually transmitted infections disproportionately affect the transgender community.[9]
  - Screen for intimate partner violence, which exists at a higher rate in the lives of transgender patients and is strongly connected to negative life outcomes.[2]
  - Substance abuse
    - Tobacco: rates of cigarette and e-cigarette use are higher in transgender populations compared with their cisgender counterparts.[10]
    - Alcohol: current data on alcohol abuse rates in transgender populations are minimal and do not provide an accurate assessment of community needs.[11]
- Mental health
  - Transgender patients have a statistically higher chance of experiencing anxiety and depression than the general population.[12] Therefore, regular assessment and counseling for psychiatric illness and suicidality are critical.

Physical

Guiding principles of the physical examination
There are several principles that should be followed throughout the physical examination to provide quality, culturally sensitive care to transgender patients.

- Anticipatory communication—before a patient is asked to undress, have an open discussion about what the physical examination will include. Explain why sensitive parts of the physical examination are important for the patient's health.
- Anatomy—physical examination should be based on the anatomy that is present, regardless of gender presentation. To this end, a sensitive history that inventories the organs and modifications present is essential.
- Language—be aware that common anatomic terminology may be distressing for transgender patients. To increase patient comfort, aim to reflect the language that the patient uses.
- Discretion and safety—only perform breast, genital, and rectal examinations when necessary. Additionally, a chaperone should be offered to the patient during sensitive examinations.[13]

Specialized components of a sensitive physical examination
- Awareness of secondary sex characteristic spectrum
  - Transfeminine patients using hormone therapy may have breast development, reduced muscle mass, reduced body hair, feminine fat distribution, softened skin, and testicles that are soft and reduced in size.[3,14]

- ○ Transmasculine patients using hormone therapy may have increased facial and body hair, acne, skin oiliness, enlarged clitoris, male pattern hair loss, deepened voice, increased upper body mass, and vaginal atrophy.[3,14]
- Transfeminine patients
  - ○ Tucking: some transfeminine patients who have not undergone genital surgery may engage in tucking.[15] Tucking of the penis and testicles can lead to complications at the external inguinal ring, such as hernias and skin breakdown.[15]
  - ○ Neovagina: a neovagina created by surgery differs from a natal vagina. It is a blind cuff with no cervix and its orientation may be more posterior. Use of an anoscope to assess vaginal walls may be preferred over a speculum.[3]
- Transmasculine patients
  - ○ Binding: many transmasculine patients who have not undergone mastectomy engage in chest binding. Complications may include skin breakdown and musculoskeletal complaints.[15] Additionally, patients may be uncomfortable removing the binding for physical examination. Counseling about safe binding practices is recommended.[15]
  - ○ Pelvic examination: some transmasculine patients may feel uncomfortable with the idea of penetration as it relates to their concept of gender, causing the pelvic examination to be especially traumatic and anxiety inducing. If a pelvic examination is indicated, special care should be taken to help patients manage this.
    - Reflect the anatomic language that the patient uses. Some transmasculine patients refer to the vaginal canal as their "front hole," whereas others prefer standard medical terminology.[3] Using a patient's preferred terminology can help reduce anxiety before and during the examination.
    - Discussion about the pelvic examination should happen while patients are fully dressed. Inquire about any past experiences with pelvic examinations, their comfort level with the examination, and what concerns they may have.[3] If patients are unduly distressed, it may be appropriate to delay the examination to a time when more rapport has been built.
    - Invite patients to use calming techniques. Some patients may prefer to bring a friend in the room, listen to music, or engage in a distracting conversation. A plan for relaxation techniques is best when discussed prior to examination.[16]
    - If anxiety cannot be managed in other ways, use of anxiolytic medications may be indicated.[16]
    - Some patients who take masculinizing hormones can experience increased discomfort during the pelvic examination due to atrophic vaginitis. This can be mitigated by administration of vaginal estrogen 1 week to 2 weeks prior to the examination.[3]

SCREENING

As outlined previously, a thorough history for transgender patients should include an organ inventory. Likewise, cancer screening should be based on the anatomy present rather than a patient's gender identity. This section outlines recommendations for cancer screening of reproductive organs, accounting for the presence or absence of gender-affirming hormones and procedures. For more on cancer in transgender patients, see Mary O. Stevenson and Vin Tangpricha's article, "Osteoporosis and Bone Health in Transgender Persons," in this issue.

Breast Cancer

Transmasculine patients

The risk of breast cancer in transmasculine patients is most powerfully stratified by top surgery, because double mastectomy substantially reduces risk.[17] The risk is not zero, however, because any residual breast tissue, including the nipple areolar complex, is at risk for the development for carcinoma.[17,18] Based on current research, there does not seem to be an increased risk of breast cancers associated with the use of gender-affirming hormone therapy.[17]

The current recommendations suggest that transmasculine patients who have not had chest surgery follow the same breast cancer screening as cisgender women.[17] For patients who have undergone bilateral mastectomy, no breast cancer screening guidelines exist.[3]

Transfeminine patients

In the cisgender female population, an association exists between hormone replacement therapy (HRT) and increased risk of breast cancer.[19] Although data are limited, this same association has not been demonstrated in the population of transfeminine patients taking gender-affirming hormone therapy.[20,21] It is known, however, that although breast cancer incidence is not increased in transfeminine patients, it does occur at younger ages (mean age of 50) than in cisgender men (mean age of 70).[20] In transfeminine patients, breast cancer also tends to present with a palpable mass.[20]

Given the earlier age of incidence of breast cancer in transfeminine patients, it is recommended that patients over the age of 50 who have used feminizing hormones for at least 5 years to 10 years have screening mammography performed every 2 years.[3] Health care providers should educate their transgender patients on the signs and symptoms of breast cancer. Mammography may be performed both on breast tissue secondary to hormonal therapy and on surgically augmented breasts.[20]

Cervical Cancer

A majority of transmasculine patients have a cervix; patients with a cervix need cervical cancer screening.[22,23] Due to dysphoria associated with the procedure, however, transmasculine patients are less likely to be up to date on cervical cancer screenings than cisgender women.[16] Screening should follow the guidelines outlined by the USPSTF, which are not modified by gender identity or hormonal therapy.[23] Cervical cancer screening is not a requirement for testosterone therapy, however, and patient refusal of screening should not be used as a barrier for hormone therapy.[3]

Ovarian Cancer

In general, routine ovarian cancer screening is not recommended for patients lacking genetic or family risk factors, and this recommendation extends to transgender patients.[24] Although exogenous testosterone therapy does change the architecture of the ovaries,[25] there is no evidence that these changes increase the risk of ovarian cancer.[3]

Some, but not all, transmasculine patients undergo single or bilateral oophorectomy for the management of gender dysphoria. Those transmasculine individuals who require pelvic imaging of ovaries but have undergone vaginectomy may receive transrectal or transabdominal ultrasound.[3]

Endometrial Cancer

Routine screening for endometrial cancer is not recommended. Exogenous testosterone therapy increases risk of endometrial atrophy, not proliferation and carcinoma.[26] For this reason, amenorrhea in these patients is not believed to increase risk of endometrial hyperplasia.[26] In the event of unexplained vaginal bleeding in the setting of testosterone-induced amenorrhea, however, the cause of bleeding should be investigated.[3]

Testicular Cancer

The USPSTF recommends against screening for testicular cancer in the general population.[27] Anatomic dysphoria, however, may pose an obstacle to early self-diagnosis of testicular cancer. Appreciation of the magnitude of anatomic dysphoria is important when interpreting patient report of symptoms.[28]

Prostate Cancer

The risks and benefits of prostate cancer screening should be discussed with all persons possessing a prostate, regardless of hormone therapy or surgical history. The prostate is not removed during feminizing surgery. The relationship between risk of prostate cancer and total testosterone has been controversial.[29] It has been historically believed that high levels of testosterone increase risk for prostate cancer and, conversely, low levels are protective. More recent studies have failed to find consistent evidence for this, however, and estrogen therapy may be less protective than once believed.[30–33] Several studies have suggested that prostate specific antigen is suppressed in the setting of low androgens and perhaps a different threshold is needed for those on antiandrogen therapies.[31,34] Because the relationship between testosterone level and prostate cancer remains unclear, prostate cancer screening should be considered for all transfeminine patients.[35]

PREVENTION
HIV

HIV prevention and education are critically important in the transgender population. Data from the Centers for Disease Control and Prevention (CDC) illustrate that HIV prevalence among transfeminine patients is the highest among all risk groups, particularly among transfeminine patients of color.[2] The rate of undiagnosed HIV in the transgender population is high—recent studies reveal that the rate of transgender patients who are undiagnosed and unaware of their HIV infection is 57% compared with a 27% national average.[9]

The foundational elements of HIV prevention include condom use and pre-exposure prophylaxis. Condom use in insertive sex can be difficult in transfeminine patients taking feminizing hormones due to reduced penile engorgement during erection.[3] Condom use in transmasculine patients with phalloplasty has not been studied. For these reasons, pre-exposure prophylaxis is be an excellent prevention choice for many transgender patients engaging in high-risk sexual behavior. There are no significant drug-drug interactions with gender affirming hormones.[36] See Lin Fraser and Gail Knudson's article, "Education Needs of Providers of Transgender Population," in this issue, for further discussion on HIV in transgender populations.

Vaccinations

The CDC recommendations for vaccinations in transgender patients do not differ from that for cisgender patients. The CDC does specifically emphasize that all young adults through the age of 26 should receive the HPV vaccine.[37] Additionally, the hepatitis B vaccine[38] is recommended particularly for those who engage in high-risk sexual behavior. Please refer to CDC guidance for the most up-to-date vaccine recommendations.

Cardiovascular Risk Reduction

Although it is well-established that supplementation of intrinsic sex hormones is linked to increases in cardiovascular disease risk, the cardiovascular risk of HRT in transgender people is poorly understood. Evidence suggests that HRT in transmasculine persons may elevate serum triglyceride and low-density lipoprotein levels while lowering high-density lipoprotein levels, although no increased risk has been demonstrated in adverse cardiovascular events.[39] In transfeminine patients, HRT has been well-documented to increase the risk of adverse cardiovascular events, specifically venous thromboembolism, myocardial infarction, and ischemic stroke. Furthermore, this risk may increase with long-term use.[39]

Some evidence suggests that transdermal estrogen may reduce the risk of venous thromboembolism in thrombophilic transfeminine patients.[40] Providers may improve the cardiovascular health of their transgender patients on HRT by encouraging smoking cessation and managing diabetes and lipid profiles.

Screening for traditional cardiovascular disease risk factors also is important.[41] Gender-affirming hormone regimens can have an impact on metabolism and affect risk of conditions like dyslipidemia and diabetes mellitus. Providers should use USPSTF recommendations and consider earlier or more frequent monitoring when eliciting a family history of premature cardiovascular disease.

Osteoporosis

Similarly, hormone regimens prescribed for transgender persons can affect bone metabolism. The traditional risk factors for osteoporosis also apply to transgender populations. Particular attention should be given to individuals postgonadectomy when hormonal regimens are discontinued.[41] A controversial area is whether or not to use assigned gender at birth when using traditional risk calculators like the Fracture Risk Assessment Tool score. A detailed discussion of bone health in transgender populations can be found elsewhere in this issue.

Contraception and Pregnancy

Transmasculine men who have not undergone hysterectomy can experience pregnancy and may have contraceptive needs. Nonhormonal options, such as condoms, are appropriate for everyone engaging in penetrative sex and have the added benefit of protection against STIs. Long-acting contraception methods that contain progesterone, such as the implant or intrauterine device, can serve a dual purpose of contraception and reduction of menstruation, especially in transmasculine patients who have recently started or are not using testosterone therapy.[42] Copper intrauterine devices are also a popular hormone-free contraceptive option, but patients should be aware that if they continue to menstruate, they can experience heavier cycles, which can exacerbate dysphoria.[43] For more on fertility considerations for transgender persons, see Michael F. Neblett II and Heather S. Hipp's article, "Fertility Considerations in Transgender Persons," in this issue.

COORDINATION OF CARE

Although transgender patients do have some unique health care needs that require specialist care, most of their health care needs overlap those of the general population and can be addressed by a primary care provider (PCP). PCPs are uniquely positioned to lead the coordination of specialist care to ensure transgender patients' health needs are being addressed comprehensively and longitudinally in an identity-affirming way. When referring to other providers, PCPs should ensure that specialists to whom they refer are gender affirming as well. Careful selection of referrals can help to prevent negative, stigmatizing experiences for transgender patients that could lead to disengagement from the health care system.[2,44]

Several nonprofit and community organizations exist that compile a list of clinics that specialize in transgender health care, including but not limited to University of California, San Francisco Center of Excellence for Transgender Health and the Trans Media Network.[3,45]

LEGAL ISSUES
Legal Identity Document Changes

Barriers to the alignment of legal documentation with gender identity stand in opposition to the physical and mental health of transgender individuals by restricting freedom of gender expression and increasing potential for harassment.[46] Health care providers are often given the role of gatekeeper for patients seeking changes to their legal identity documents, and thus it is imperative physicians stay abreast of current regulatory matters to provide the best care and guidance for their transgender patients.

Although there are efforts to make laws consistent across the nation, matters of amending legal identity documents depend on an intricate mix of both federal and state laws.

Federal documents

To change legal gender, a health professional must certify, in writing, that the patient has undergone "necessary" medical or psychological treatment for transition.[44,45] Currently, no particular clinical treatment, including hormones and surgery, has been determined necessary for all transgender patients, possibly opening the door to interpretation by individual providers.[3] The following United States federal bodies have adopted similar rules regarding changes to identity documents:

- Department of State, for issuing passports and consular birth certificates
- Social Security Administration
- Department of Homeland Security
- Veterans Health Administration
- Office of Personnel Management[47]

State documents

Many states fall in line with federal law; however, some require surgical intervention to change legal gender. As with the case of federal law, no specific surgery has been established as necessary for all transgender patients, leaving flexibility in interpretation by the provider.[3]

- Birth certificate: changing legal gender on a birth certificate is complex because this document is considered a vital record and accepted as official by many agencies. Birth certificates are administered through local and territorial jurisdictions and many require a court order and/or documentation from a surgeon confirming gender-affirming surgery to amend them. Several jurisdictions, however, have eliminated surgical requirements completely. Few states currently forbid or prohibit correction of gender designation on birth certificates.[48]
- Driver's license: driver's license changes depend on the state of residence. Departments of motor vehicles in approximately half of the states have removed surgical requirements for gender marker corrections.[48]
- Name change: in most jurisdictions, the legal name change procedure for transgender individuals is identical to that for nontransgender people because this is a nongendered process.[47]

Once legal documents have been amended, it is important that legal name and gender are updated with insurance companies and medical providers to prevent denial of claims based on a mismatch of legal gender and gender-specific medical care. Providers may be required to contact the insurance company and advocate for their patient in circumstances of gender-specific denial.[3]

Legal Considerations for Minors

- Document changes: individuals under the age of 18 must have parental consent to change their legal name or gender marker on government identification. This process varies by state.
- Gender-affirming therapy: initiation of prescription hormone therapy has no set age limit and is up to the health provider's discretion. Both gonadotropin-releasing hormone analog and gender-affirming hormone administration require parental or guardian consent if a patient is under the age of 18.[3] For more on hormone therapy in minors, see Jessica Abramowitz's article, "Hormone Therapy in Children and Adolescents," in this issue.
- Parental consent challenges: if parents or guardians of transgender children have conflicting opinions about initiating gender-affirming therapy and maintaining medical decision-making power, then it becomes the task of the mental and medical health providers to educate the parents or guardians on the necessity of medical intervention. In the case of transgender youth in the child welfare system, judges are permitted to order medical intervention, including gender-affirming hormone therapy.[3]

Resources

The National Center for Transgender Equality, TransLine: Transgender Medical Consultation Service managed by Project HEALTH, and Lambda Legal maintain updated guidance on federal and state-specific regulations for changing legal identity documents.

SUMMARY

The preventive health care needs of transgender patients differ minimally from the remainder of the population. For this reason, any health care provider with a sensitive approach and proper training can feel confident in caring for this population.

There are several key recommendations that any provider can implement to improve the experience of transgender patients in the health care setting:

- Providers should ensure that the entirety of the patient encounter is adaptable and sensitive to the needs of transgender patients. To this end, clinics should provide staff with sensitivity training and ensure the adaptability of EHRs.
- During the clinical encounter, PCPs should conduct a history and physical examination as they would with any patient, specifically emphasizing considerations of patient privacy, transparency, and cultural sensitivity.
- Review of systems, physical examination, and cancer screenings should be based on a patient's existing anatomy rather than gender identity. In addition to individual patients' risk factors, preventive health discussions should consider the transgender population's increased risk for HIV as well as the influence of gender-affirming hormones on cardiovascular health. Further investigation is required to better understand cancer risks in patients taking gender-affirming hormones.

- Providers should always maintain LGBTQ+-friendly referral lists in the event that patients need specialized care.
- Finally, health care providers should keep in mind the important role they may play in their patients' legal gender transitions, keeping themselves abreast of major laws and regulations in the state in which they practice.

REFERENCES

1. James SE, Herman JL, Rankin S, et al. The report of the 2015 U.S. Transgender Survey. Washington, DC: National Center for Transgender Equality; 2016.
2. National LGBTQ Task Force. Injustice at every turn: a report of the national transgender discrimination survey. 2011. Available at: http://www.thetaskforce.org/injustice-every-turn-report-national-transgender-discrimination-survey/. Accessed September 5, 2018.
3. Guidelines for the Primary and Gender-Affirming Care of Transgender and Gender Nonbinary People. 2016.
4. Gay & Lesbian Medical Association. Guidelines for care of lesbian, gay, bisexual, and transgender patients. Available at: https://npin.cdc.gov/publication/guidelines-care-lesbian-gay-bisexual-and-transgender-patients. Accessed September 13, 2018.
5. Torres CG, Renfrew M, Kenst K, et al. Improving transgender health by building safe clinical environments that promote existing resilience: Results from a qualitative analysis of providers. BMC Pediatr 2015;15:187.
6. Deutsch MB, Green J, Keatley J, et al. Electronic medical records and the transgender patient: recommendations from the World Professional Association for Transgender Health EMR Working Group. J Am Med Inform Assoc 2013;20(4): 700-3.
7. Wallace PM, Rasmussen S. Analysis of adulterated silicone: implications for health promotion. Int J Transgend 2010;12(3):167-75.
8. Wilczynski C, Emanuele MA. Treating a transgender patient: overview of the guidelines. Postgrad Med 2014;126(7):121-8.
9. Sevelius JM, Keatley J, Gutierrez-Mock L. HIV/AIDS programming in the United States: considerations affecting transgender women and girls. Womens Health Issues 2011;21(6 Suppl):S278-82.
10. Hoffman L, Delahanty J, Johnson SE, et al. Sexual and gender minority cigarette smoking disparities: an analysis of 2016 behavioral risk factor surveillance system data. Prev Med 2018;113:109-15.
11. Gilbert PA, Pass LE, Keuroghlian AS, et al. Alcohol research with transgender populations: a systematic review and recommendations to strengthen future studies. Drug Alcohol Depend 2018;186:138-46.
12. Budge SL, Adelson JL, Howard KAS. Anxiety and depression in transgender individuals: the roles of transition status, loss, social support, and coping. J Consult Clin Psychol 2013;81(3):545-57.
13. Tollinche LE, Walters CB, Radix A, et al. The perioperative care of the transgender patient. Anesth Analg 2018;127(2):359-66.
14. Feldman JL, Goldberg JM. Transgender primary medical care. International Journal of Transgenderism 2006;9.3-4:3-34.
15. Binding, packing, tucking & padding. Available at: http://www.phsa.ca/transcarebc/care-support/transitioning/bind-pack-tuck-pad. Accessed September 7, 2018.

16. Peitzmeier SM, Khullar K, Reisner SL, et al. Pap test use is lower among female-to-male patients than non-transgender women. Am J Prev Med 2014;47(6): 808–12.

17. Stone JP, Hartley RL, Temple-Oberle C. Breast cancer in transgender patients: a systematic review. Part 2: female to male. Eur J Surg Oncol 2018. https://doi.org/10.1016/j.ejso.2018.06.021.

18. Shao T, Grossbard ML, Klein P. Breast cancer in female-to-male transsexuals: two cases with a review of physiology and management. Clin Breast Cancer 2011; 11(6):417–9.

19. Rossouw JE, Anderson GL, Prentice RL, et al, Writing Group for the Women's Health Initiative Investigators. Risks and benefits of estrogen plus progestin in healthy postmenopausal women: principal results from the women's health initiative randomized controlled trial. JAMA 2002;288(3):321–33.

20. Hartley RL, Stone JP, Temple-Oberle C. Breast cancer in transgender patients: A systematic review. Part 1: male to female. Eur J Surg Oncol 2018. https://doi.org/10.1016/j.ejso.2018.06.035.

21. Asscheman H, Giltay EJ, Megens JAJ, et al. A long-term follow-up study of mortality in transsexuals receiving treatment with cross-sex hormones. Eur J Endocrinol 2011;164(4):635–42.

22. Gatos KC. A literature review of cervical cancer screening in transgender men. Nurs Womens Health 2018;22(1):52–62.

23. Final update summary: cervical cancer: screening - US preventive services task force. Available at: https://www.uspreventiveservicestaskforce.org/Page/Document/UpdateSummaryFinal/cervical-cancer-screening2. Accessed September 5, 2018.

24. Screening for ovarian cancer: US preventive services task force recommendation statement | Cancer screening, prevention, control | JAMA | JAMA Network. Available at: https://jamanetwork-com.proxy.library.emory.edu/journals/jama/fullarticle/2672638. Accessed September 5, 2018.

25. Grynberg M, Fanchin R, Dubost G, et al. Histology of genital tract and breast tissue after long-term testosterone administration in a female-to-male transsexual population. Reprod Biomed Online 2010;20(4):553–8.

26. Perrone AM, Cerpolini S, Salfi NCM, et al. Effect of long-term testosterone administration on the endometrium of female-to-male (FtM) transsexuals. J Sex Med 2009;6(11):3193–200.

27. Final update summary: testicular cancer: screening - US preventive services task force. Available at: https://www.uspreventiveservicestaskforce.org/Page/Document/UpdateSummaryFinal/testicular-cancer-screening. Accessed September 5, 2018.

28. Dhand A, Dhaliwal G. Examining patient conceptions: a case of metastatic breast cancer in an African American male to female transgender patient. J Gen Intern Med 2010;25(2):158–61.

29. Klap J, Schmid M, Loughlin KR. The relationship between total testosterone levels and prostate cancer: a review of the continuing controversy. J Urol 2015;193(2): 403–14.

30. Morgentaler A. Testosterone and prostate cancer: an historical perspective on a modern myth. Eur Urol 2006;50(5):935–9.

31. Morgentaler A, Bruning CO, DeWolf WC. Occult prostate cancer in men with low serum testosterone levels. JAMA 1996;276(23):1904–6.

32. Turo R, Jallad S, Prescott S, et al. Metastatic prostate cancer in transsexual diagnosed after three decades of estrogen therapy. Can Urol Assoc J 2013;7(7–8): E544–6.

33. Morgentaler A. Testosterone deficiency and prostate cancer: emerging recognition of an important and troubling relationship. Eur Urol 2007;52(3):623–5.

34. Gooren L, Morgentaler A. Prostate cancer incidence in orchidectomised male-to-female transsexual persons treated with oestrogens. Andrologia 2014;46(10): 1156–60.

35. Deebel NA, Morin JP, Autorino R, et al. Prostate cancer in transgender women: incidence, etiopathogenesis, and management challenges. Urology 2017;110: 166–71.

36. Pre-Exposure Prophylaxis (PrEP) | HIV Risk and Prevention | HIV/AIDS | CDC. 2018. Available at: https://www.cdc.gov/hiv/risk/prep/index.html. Accessed September 7, 2018.

37. HPV Vaccine Recommendations | Human Papillomavirus | CDC. 2017. Available at: https://www.cdc.gov/vaccines/vpd/hpv/hcp/recommendations. html. Accessed September 21, 2018.

38. Schillie S. Prevention of hepatitis B virus infection in the United States: recommendations of the advisory committee on immunization practices. MMWR Recomm Rep 2018;67. https://doi.org/10.15585/mmwr.rr6701a1.

39. Maraka S, Singh Ospina N, Rodriguez-Gutierrez R, et al. Sex steroids and cardiovascular outcomes in transgender individuals: a systematic review and meta-analysis. J Clin Endocrinol Metab 2017;102(11):3914–23.

40. Getahun D, Nash R, Flanders WD, et al. Cross-sex hormones and acute cardiovascular events in transgender persons: a cohort study. Ann Intern Med 2018. https://doi.org/10.7326/M17-2785.

41. Hembree WC, Cohen-Kettenis PT, Gooren L, et al. endocrine treatment of gender-dysphoric/gender-incongruent persons: an endocrine society clinical practice guideline. J Clin Endocrinol Metab 2017;102(11):3869–903.

42. Light A, Wang L-F, Zeymo A, et al. Family planning and contraception use in transgender men. Contraception 2018;98(4):266–9.

43. Bentsianov S, Gordon L, Goldman A, et al. Use of copper intrauterine device in transgender male adolescents. Contraception 2018;98(1):74–5.

44. McNair RP, Hegarty K. Guidelines for the primary care of lesbian, gay, and bisexual people: a systematic review. Ann Fam Med 2010;8(6):533–41.

45. Trans Media Network. Trans Health Clinics. Trans Health. Available at: http://www. trans-health.com/clinics/. Accessed September 6, 2018.

46. World Professional Association for Transgender Health. WPATH 2017 Identity Recognition Statement. 2017. Available at: https://tgeu.org/wpath-2017-identity-recognition-statement/. Accessed September 5, 2018.

47. National Center for Transgender Equality. ID Documents Center. Available at: https://transequality.org/documents. Accessed September 5, 2018.

48. TransLine: Transgender Medical Consultation Service. Changing Identity Documents. Available at: https://transline.zendesk.com/hc/en-us/categories/ 204101227-Changing-Identity-Documents. Accessed September 8, 2018.

Fertility Considerations in Transgender Persons

Michael F. Neblett II, MD[a], Heather S. Hipp, MD[b],*

KEYWORDS

- Fertility preservation • Transgender • Sperm • Oocyte • Embryo • Cryopreservation
- Adolescents

KEY POINTS

- The desire for transgender persons to have children is the same as cis-gender individuals, and many would strongly consider fertility preservation if presented with the opportunity.
- Hormone and surgical therapy frequently used for gender affirmation have significant repercussions for future fertility.
- Current fertility preservation options include sperm cryopreservation for transwomen and oocyte or embryo cryopreservation for transmen.
- Current experimental options for prepubertal transgender adolescents include testicular and ovarian tissue cryopreservation.
- Physicians should counsel and discuss fertility preservation options to transgender persons, ideally before undergoing hormone therapy or gender affirmation surgery.

INTRODUCTION

Gender-affirming therapy, including gonadectomy (removal of testes or ovaries) and exogenous hormone therapy, is a medically necessary treatment to alleviate gender dysphoria; both, however, can result in loss of reproductive potential. Discussing fertility preservation before initiation of hormonal or surgical treatment provides patients the opportunity to preserve gametes for future use via cryopreservation of sperm, oocytes, embryos, or reproductive tissue. Historically, fertility preservation has been used in oncofertility with the purpose of maximizing the reproductive potential of patients with cancer before medical treatment that may cause infertility, such as radiation therapy or chemotherapy. This emerging field, however, provides an

Disclosure Statement: The authors have no nothing to disclose.
[a] Department of Gynecology and Obstetrics, Emory University, Emory University School of Medicine, Glenn Building, 4th Floor–412 B, 69 Jesse Hill Jr. Drive Southeast, Atlanta, GA 30303, USA; [b] Division of Reproductive Endocrinology and Infertility, Department of Gynecology and Obstetrics, Emory University School of Medicine, 550 Peachtree Street, Suite 1800, Atlanta, GA 30308, USA
* Corresponding author.
E-mail address: hhipp@emory.edu

Endocrinol Metab Clin N Am 48 (2019) 391–402
https://doi.org/10.1016/j.ecl.2019.02.003
0889-8529/19/© 2019 Elsevier Inc. All rights reserved.

endo.theclinics.com

excellent opportunity to offer education and treatment aimed at protecting future reproductive ability for transgender patients.

The desire for transgender persons to have children is the same as for cis-gender individuals, because 50% to 58% of transgender patients desire future children and 37% to 76% would consider fertility preservation.[1,2] However, 1 large multicenter study of 189 transgender people in Germany found that only 9.6% of transwomen and 3.1% of transmen had actually undergone fertility preservation.[1] Common barriers include infrequent counseling, undesired side effects of endogenous hormones, sometimes invasive procedures, and delay or cessation of hormones or surgery.

There are currently no practice guidelines for physicians providing fertility preservation, and there are limited studies to guide reproductive care to transgender persons. The World Professional Association for Transgender Health, The Endocrine Society, and The American Society for Reproductive Medicine (ASRM) recommend and agree that, before starting hormone therapy or undergoing surgery to remove or alter their reproductive organs, individuals should be counseled about the effect of treatment on their fertility.[3–5] More than 90% of the US population agree with or were neutral to physicians providing fertility care to transgender individuals.[6] Even with this recommendation, transgender patients continue to face discrimination and confusion from providers and receive substandard care resulting in difficulty accessing fertility preservation services.[7] This substandard care includes the failure of most health insurance plans to cover the cost of mental health services, hormone therapy, or gender affirmation surgery. The American College of Obstetricians and Gynecologists opposes discrimination on the basis of gender dysphoria and urges physicians to eliminate barriers for improved access to care.[8]

The goal of this review is to discuss medical treatment effects on fertility, available and experimental options of fertility preservation for transgender persons, and strategies for improved care.

MEDICAL TREATMENT EFFECTS ON FERTILITY

Hormonal therapy with or without gender confirmation surgery is a common approach to alleviate gender dysphoria and allow for transgender persons to live successfully in desired gender roles. The 2 major goals of hormonal therapy are to first, reduce endogenous hormone levels to suppress secondary sex characteristics of the individual's sex designated at birth, and, second, to replace endogenous sex hormones levels with those of the affirmed gender identity using hormone replacement treatment (either estrogen or testosterone).[4] The physical changes associated with sex hormone transitioning are usually accompanied by improvement in mental well-being, but are often at the expense of future fertility. Furthermore, although it may be important to have the option of a biological child, the idea of stopping hormones or having a feminizing experience of pregnancy is often not of interest.[9]

Thresholds have not yet been established for the amount and duration of exogenous estrogen or testosterone necessary to have a permanent negative effect on fertility. In addition, for an improved physical appearance, surgery on several body areas is sometimes pursued, with the most important being gonadectomy. Loss of reproductive potential is easier to understand after surgical removal of gonads with irreversible damage to reproductive organs, but changes are less clear with hormonal therapy. This section discusses the role of gender hormones and the effect on future fertility.

The hormone regimen for transwomen typically includes use of antiandrogens in conjunction with estrogen. Antiandrogens have been shown to be effective in reducing endogenous testosterone levels while allowing estrogen to have its fullest effect.[4] The most common antiandrogen used in the United States is spironolactone, which directly inhibits androgen secretion and inhibits androgen binding to the androgen receptor.[10] Estrogen is the fundamental component for feminization in transwomen and can be given via oral, transdermal, or parenteral route, with goal estradiol levels of 100 to 200 pg/mL.[4]

In transgender women, research suggests that prolonged estrogen exposure of the testes has been associated with testicular damage.[4] Estrogen exposure can suppress androgen production and spermatogenesis. In 1 study of orchiectomy specimens, long-term exposure to estrogen caused aspermatogenesis with maturation arrest in 80% of people and hypospermatogenesis with focal spermatid/mature spermatozoa in 20% of people.[11] Long-term exposure to estrogen also causes a significant decrease in the diameter of seminiferous tubules and fatty degeneration of surrounding connective tissue with absence or reduction in the number of Leydig cells.[12,13] Additional suggested histologic changes include rare cytomegaly and epididymal hyperplasia.[11] Of note, however, a recent review of 11 publications found heterogeneous histologic analyses in orchiectomy specimens, from normal spermatogenesis to full testicular regression with severe cellular damage.[14]

Sperm concentration in the ejaculate and restoration of spermatogenesis following extended estrogen treatment have not been well studied. One study of a eugonadal man who received 2 different regimens of treatment with ethinyl estradiol showed varying semen parameters with dose of estrogen.[15] Low-dose estrogen had no negative effect on sperm motility and density for approximately 4 weeks. With high doses, reduced motility was noted after a few days with a significant decrease in sperm concentration after 2 weeks. After stopping estrogen, motility returned to normal values quicker than concentration, with pretherapeutic normal values obtained after 70 days after low-dose and 100 days after high-dose estrogen. Further studies to delineate time of sperm return to the ejaculate following cessation of hormone therapy have not been published.

In transmen, testosterone is the key hormone that acts directly on end organs to induce male secondary sex characteristics. Either parenteral or transdermal preparations can be used to achieve testosterone values in the normal male range, typically 320 to 1000 ng/dL.[4] The effects of prolonged treatment of exogenous testosterone on ovarian function are unclear. Testosterone therapy leads to an anovulatory state and amenorrhea that is usually reversible upon discontinuation of testosterone therapy.[16] Cessation of menses on average occurs within 3 months of therapy initiation,[17] but can occur as late as 8 to 12 months[16] or as soon as 1 month with high doses of testosterone.[18]

Testosterone exposure has known influences on ovarian tissue. Anti-Mullerian hormone (AMH), a marker for ovarian reserve, is significantly lower after androgenic therapy; 1 study found a decrease in mean AMH from 4.4 ng/mL to 1.4 ng/mL after initiation of testosterone and an aromatase inhibitor.[19] This suppression was noted over a short period of 16 weeks. In a study of 11 transmen with regular cycles before initiation of prolonged testosterone, evaluation of ovaries histologically at time of gender confirmation surgery showed stromal hyperplasia and luteinization, thickened ovarian cortex, and accelerated follicular atresia as compared with controls.[20] Follicular arrest was confirmed in another study of 40 transmen following testosterone treatment whose ovaries were examined; most of the follicles were primordial (60%) or intermediate (27%) with a very low number of secondary follicles (1.3%). The distribution of the follicles within the cortex, however, appeared similar to controls.[21] Interestingly, follicular development (or lack thereof) was unrelated to serum testosterone levels.

Testosterone can also have an effect on the uterine endometrium, potentially affecting implantation. Testosterone is known to bind to androgen receptors in the endometrium and cause a predominant atrophic effect.[16,22] However, it has also been suggested that long-term testosterone use could cause a proliferative effect on endometrial tissue, even raising the risk of hyperplasia. Tangential but related to fertility, there are no guidelines regarding endometrial surveillance currently for transmen on testosterone. Any abnormal uterine bleeding should be investigated with pathologic endometrial evaluation.

REPRODUCTIVE OPTIONS FOR TRANSGENDER WOMEN

The best option for fertility preservation for transwomen is cryopreservation of sperm before initiation of hormone therapy or gender confirmation surgery. Cryopreservation refers to the cooling of cells and tissues to subzero temperatures in order to stop all biologic activity and preserve them for future use.[23] As noted above, estrogen has significant deleterious effects on sperm production. Fertility preservation after beginning hormone therapy does necessitate stopping hormones, which may lead to undesirable side effects of increased endogenous testosterone production. However, fertility preservation can still be offered anytime during transitioning. Recommendations regarding length of time off hormones for return of ejaculation and sperm presence are unclear, but, as suggested earlier, longer time on hormones has worsening effects on semen parameters.

Sperm cryopreservation is the technique of sperm preservation with a sample typically obtained through masturbation. Collecting sperm via masturbation is usually simple but can be a difficult burden to transwomen.[24] If hormone therapy has already been initiated, there can also be difficulty with erection and ejaculation. Potential collection aids include penile vibratory stimulation (PVS) and electroejaculation (EEJ), which can be used to obtain sperm, similarly to men with spinal cord injuries.[25] With PVS, a vibrator is placed at the tip of the penis to facilitate ejaculation. With EEJ, an electric probe is inserted into the rectum, typically with anesthesia. Electrical stimulation is used to elicit ejaculation using increasing frequency and amplitude. Sperm can additionally be retrieved directly from the testis or epididymis via surgical sperm retrieval; however, these procedures are very invasive and infrequently used when not in the context of male factor infertility. They can be performed at the time of testes removal with gender-affirming surgery.

Excellent-quality sperm can be used for intrauterine insemination (IUI), in which sperm are directly deposited into the uterus of the partner with a catheter at the time of ovulation. Best results are obtained with at least 10 million motile sperm in each IUI; however, there is still a reasonable chance of success if 5 million motile sperm are present.[26] To reach these concentrations, it may be necessary for a person to collect multiple times to bank sperm to make IUI feasible. In addition, depending on the age of the partner, each IUI only has approximately 10% chance of success; multiple cycles may be necessary. Sperm of poor or limited quantity can be used for in vitro fertilization (IVF) with intracytoplasmic sperm injection (ICSI), which is discussed later.

An overview of fertility preservation options in transwomen is shown in **Table 1**. Testicular tissue cryopreservation is still considered experimental and discussed later in the child and adolescent section. Last, several recently reported cases of uterine transplantation into nontransgender women represent a potential future reproductive option; however, this technology is still in the beginning stages of research.[27]

REPRODUCTIVE OPTIONS FOR TRANSGENDER MEN

Fertility preservation options for transmen include oocyte cryopreservation, embryo cryopreservation, and ovarian tissue cryopreservation (OTC), which is still

Table 1
Summary of current fertility preservation options for transgender persons

Method	Description	Status	Considerations
Transwomen			
Sperm Cryopreservation	Cryopreservation of sperm obtained via masturbation, assisted ejaculation, or surgically extracted from testis or epididymis	Established method	Future uses include IUI or IVF with ICSI depending on quantity and quality of sperm retrieved
Testicular tissue cryopreservation	Cryopreservation of testicular tissue after surgical biopsy with cryopreservation/transplantation of spermatogonium stem cells	Experimental	Prepubertal or postpubertal, possible removal at time of gender affirmation surgery
Transmen			
Oocyte cryopreservation	Hormonal stimulation followed by ultrasound-guided retrieval of oocytes with vitrification of unfertilized oocytes. Can be thawed and fertilized later to create embryos in future	Established method	Sperm is not required, stress from hormonal side effects, repeat pelvic examinations, TVUS, and retrieval process
Embryo cryopreservation	Hormonal stimulation followed by ultrasound-guided retrieval of oocytes with fertilization (conventional vs ICSI) to form embryos that are cryopreserved for future use	Established method	Sperm is required, which has ethical concerns Stress from hormonal side effects, repeat pelvic examinations, TVUS, and retrieval process
Ovarian Tissue Cryopreservation	Removal and cryopreservation of the outer layer of ovary (cortex), which contains oocytes, or entire ovary	Experimental	Prepubertal or postpubertal, ovarian tissue usually obtained via outpatient laparoscopic approach, reimplanted into the pelvis (orthotopic), or arm/abdominal wall (heterotopic)
In vitro maturation	Oocytes are retrieved and then matured in vitro to achieve fertilization and embryo development outside the body	Experimental	Prepubertal or postpubertal, less unwanted hormonal side effects

experimental in the United States. These techniques are more invasive and present a greater challenge for fertility preservation because cryopreservation of oocytes or embryos are obtained via controlled ovarian hyperstimulation cycles and subsequent oocyte retrieval, a process that typically takes 2 weeks. Injectable gonadotropins are given daily to stimulate growth of multiple ovarian follicles, while, at the same time, gonadotropin releasing hormone (GnRH) agonist or antagonist is given to down-regulate the pituitary gland to prevent premature ovulation. During ovarian stimulation, there are frequent transvaginal ultrasounds (TVUS) to assess the growth of follicles along with blood draws for serum estradiol and progesterone levels. When the follicles have reached the appropriate size and oocyte maturation is triggered, oocytes are collected approximately 36 hours later via ultrasound-guided transvaginal aspiration. Mature oocytes can be cryopreserved. If embryo cryopreservation is desired, oocytes are next fertilized. Sperm can be provided by an intimate partner or from a known or anonymous sperm donor. The embryos can then be used for establishing a pregnancy using the patient's uterus or by transfer into a partner or gestational carrier's uterus.

Embryo cryopreservation has conventionally been used as a means of fertility preservation and yields reliable pregnancy outcomes. However, sperm is needed, which may raise ethical, religious, and legal concerns regarding future use. With improved pregnancy rates and outcomes over time, the experimental label from oocyte cryopreservation was removed in 2012 by the ASRM.[23] Vitrification, a method of rapidly cooling cells without ice crystal formation, improves oocyte survival rates and offers comparable pregnancy rates of those of fresh oocytes.[23] ASRM specified that outcome data at the time of publication were restricted to oocyte donors and infertile couples, but that it could be offered to women before gonadotoxic treatment (eg, chemotherapy), women at high risk for primary ovarian insufficiency or for oophorectomy, or in couples who do not have sperm available at the time of retrieval. Transgender people were not included in the ASRM committee opinion; however, this technology offers transmen the option of improved autonomy over their gametes, because no sperm is required at time of decision to undergo cryopreservation, and they can use donor sperm in the future if desired. No increases in chromosomal abnormalities, birth defects, or developmental deficits have been noted in the children born from cryopreserved oocytes as compared with IVF pregnancies.[23] Importantly, for oocytes to be used in the future, they must be thawed and fertilized with sperm, and the subsequent embryo or embryos cultured in the laboratory and then transferred to a uterus.

The chances of pregnancy with IVF (using fresh or frozen oocytes) are highly dependent on the age of the oocyte, with declining rates with advancing age.[28] In addition to age, a larger number of oocytes or embryos cryopreserved results in higher chance of a successful live birth; 1 study recommended cryopreserving at least 15 to 20 oocytes for a 70% to 80% chance of live birth in patients under 38 years of age.[29]

Since 2012, there have been some data published in the transgender population. In 2014, the first transman underwent oocyte cryopreservation at age 17 before initiating androgen therapy.[30] Since that time, pregnancy outcomes have been reported after cryopreservation of oocytes in transmen with transfer of oocytes to cis-gender female partners.[31] This field is an exciting and upcoming field of fertility preservations, and further data are needed for improved discussion of outcomes. An overview of fertility preservation options in transmen is shown in **Table 1**. OTC is still considered experimental and is discussed later.

Transmen who do desire fertility preservation through oocyte or embryo cryopreservation need to temporarily stop taking hormone therapy, which can present a significant barrier. The amount of time off of testosterone is not well studied. Anecdotal reports from fertility clinics report recommendations of 1 to 6 months off of testosterone for its effect on the ovaries to wane. In addition, time off of testosterone and the ovarian stimulation regimens increase serum estrogen levels, which can lead to unwanted physical changes and resumption of menstrual bleeding.[32] These changes can cause a great deal of stress and gender dysphoria in patients. To avoid high levels of estrogen effects during stimulation and improved patient compliance, a stimulation protocol with the addition of an aromatase inhibitor can also be considered,[33] although this application has been studied primarily in patients with estrogen-sensitive cancers.[34] Other potential stresses from oocyte/embryo cryopreservation cycles include need for pelvic examinations, frequent TVUS, and the actual retrieval procedure itself.[35] Some suggested coping strategies from a recent review include "focus on the reason the patient is undergoing fertility preservation, recommend reaching out to supportive family or friends, using transabdominal ultrasound monitoring if body mass index allows, using nongendered names of body parts, and sensitivity training for medical personnel on use of appropriate pronouns."[35]

Unfortunately, assisted reproductive options are expensive and frequently not covered by insurance companies.[32] Mental health counseling by an educated counselor and support from a multidisciplinary team should also be made available for transgender patients pursuing reproductive options.[36]

PREGNANCY OUTCOMES IN TRANSGENDER MEN

For transmen who do wish to conceive, there has been some literature published regarding pregnancies in this population following prolonged testosterone treatment. Although these data are lacking, transmen who have initiated transitioning have been able to discontinue testosterone therapy to undergo insemination of sperm or embryo transfer to establish a pregnancy. In a study of 25 transmen who experienced pregnancy after the use of testosterone, 20 resumed menses within 6 months of stopping testosterone and 5 were still amenorrheic at time of conception.[37] Twenty-one pregnancies were from the patient's own gonads (ovaries). Obstetric outcomes were similar in the patients who had previously taken testosterone and those who had not. One important finding of this study was that a third of the pregnancies were unplanned, highlighting the need to discuss contraception and family planning because many transmen retain their reproductive organs and capacity to have children. This counseling should also include a discussion of stopping testosterone if trying to conceive and during pregnancy. In addition, further discussion should be made regarding anticipating increasing gender dysphoria during pregnancy, routine obstetric care, mode and environment of delivery, and postpartum considerations, including options for infant feeding and when to reinitiate testosterone.[38]

FERTILITY PRESERVATION OPTIONS FOR CHILDREN AND ADOLESCENTS

With increasing attention on and care about transgender issues in the past decade, more transgender children and adolescents are seeking pubertal suppression and treatment with gender-affirming hormones. Before initiation, they and their guardians should be counseled regarding options for fertility preservation. This exciting and expanding field can be controversial among providers and an opportunity for further education and research. The rates of fertility preservation utilization among transgender youth have been shown to be low, at only 3% to 4% in 2 recent studies.[39,40]

A significant ethical concern regarding fertility preservation among transgender youth is that parents must decide and make decisions regarding fertility preservation before initiation of pubertal suppression and/or gender-affirming hormone therapy.

Although ideally these decisions are made with input from the youth, they may not fully understand the implications of their present decisions.[3,4] This potential discord between an adolescent and their parent results in parental decisions that may not fully align with future desires and may set up disagreements and tension between parents and youth. To alleviate some of this stress, many physicians follow Endocrine Society recommendations and offer pubertal suppression using GnRH analogues until age 16.[4] GnRH agonists prevent development of secondary sex characteristics and suspend germ cell maturation that is usually reversible and should not impair resumption of puberty upon cessation.[41] The GnRH agonist allows time for the adolescent to work with a mental health therapist to explore options and live in the experienced gender role. However, most children do begin gender-affirming hormone therapy without undergoing puberty.[4]

In children who have undergone puberty, fertility preservation options are the same as previously described in the adult, including sperm, oocyte, and embryo cryopreservation. However, it is not yet possible for youth who have not undergone puberty to undergo fertility preservation to preserve gametes with the current standard care. There are experimental options that are not yet widely available but may present a future option as live births have been reported.

For transgender girls who have not yet undergone spermarche, testicular tissue cryopreservation and spermatogonium stem cell transplantation are potential options; however, both are still considered experimental. Spermarche is an early pubertal event with a median age of 13.4 years old and can occur before development of pubic hair or testicular growth.[42] It is reasonable to attempt masturbation and sperm collection even in younger adolescents if testicular volume is greater than 5 mL.[43] Testicular tissue cryopreservation is still under investigation, but current research is being undertaken in oncology patients and adolescents.[44,45] Prepubertally, testicular tissue contains spermatogonium, which are male germ cells located in seminiferous tubules; eventually, these undergo spermatogenesis to form mature sperm. Cryopreservation of the spermatogonium stem cells, followed by transplantation into the testis or in vitro maturation to produce sperm to use for ICSI/IVF, is a proposed clinical option for fertility preservation. No pregnancies in humans have been reported to date.[45,46]

For transgender boys, OTC is currently the only fertility preservation option and is still considered an experimental procedure by ASRM.[47] Of note, however, there have been several case series of live births reported worldwide resulting after autotransplantation of cryopreserved ovarian tissue. These series were in patients with prior cancer with treatment requiring chemotherapy and/or radiation.[48,49] In a case series of 49 women who were followed more than 1 year after autotransplantation, the ovaries were active in 67% of the women, and pregnancy and delivery rates were noted to be 33% and 25%, respectively.[50] In 2015, the first report of a live birth after autograft of OTC before menarche was reported, which offered evidence for a potential means of fertility preservation in prepubertal transgender boys.[51]

The technique of OTC includes biopsies of ovarian cortex or removal of the entire ovary, cryopreservation until fertility is desired, tissue thawing, and then reimplantation back into the body.[47] Ovarian tissue is most commonly obtained via a laparoscopic approach, but a minilaparotomy may be needed in select cases. The outer layer of the ovary, or ovarian cortex, which contains most oocytes, is then sectioned into thin pieces and cryopreserved via slow freeze or vitrification. Ideally, this process is started before initiation of hormone therapy but has been performed after sustained androgen exposure.[21] The ovarian tissue sections are later reimplanted into the pelvis (orthotopic) or arm/abdominal wall (heterotopic) during a second procedure. Orthotopic reimplantation is more common, and currently has better outcomes than a heterotopic approach.[47]

Reimplantation of ovarian tissue in transmen not only restores ovarian function to produce oocytes but additionally restores endocrine function with potentially un-wanted hormone side effects. In an effort to combat these side effects, 1 potential op-tion is in vitro maturation, in which oocytes are retrieved and then matured in vitro to achieve fertilization and embryo development outside the body. This experimental procedure is still in early research but offers a unique role in fertility preservation because live births have been reported.[52]

SUMMARY

Hormone therapy and/or gender affirmation surgery to alleviate gender dysphoria in transgender patients can have a devastating effect on reproductive potential. Fertility preservation is an important topic to discuss with transgender patients, and multiple organizations agree that physicians ideally should have this conversation before initi-ation of hormone or surgical therapy. With adolescents, care should be taken to incor-porate guardians for a collaborative discussion.

Studies have shown that transgender persons have the same desire to have chil-dren as cis-gender individuals, and many would strongly consider fertility preservation if asked. However, transgender patients receive infrequent counseling and limited ac-cess to treatment of fertility preservation. In addition, there are currently no practice guidelines for physicians providing reproductive care to transgender patients. Fertility preservation for transgender persons is an emerging field that requires further research, collaboration between providers, development of guidelines, improved education, and counseling to patients.

REFERENCES

1. Auer MK, Fuss J, Nieder TO, et al. Desire to have children among transgender people in germany: a cross-sectional multi-center study. J Sex Med 2018;15(5): 757–67.
2. Wierckx K, Van Caenegem E, Pennings G, et al. Reproductive wish in transsexual men. Hum Reprod 2012;27(2):483–7.
3. Standards of care for the health of transsexual, transgender,and gender noncon-forming people. 7th edition. World Professional Association for Transgender Health; 2011. Available at: https://www.wpath.org/publications/soc.
4. Hembree WC, Cohen-Kettenis PT, Gooren L, et al. Endocrine treatment of gender-dysphoric/gender-incongruent persons: an endocrine society clinical practice guideline. J Clin Endocrinol Metab 2017;102(11):3869–903.
5. Martinez F. Update on fertility preservation from the barcelona international soci-ety for fertility preservation-ESHRE-ASRM 2015 expert meeting: indications, re-sults and future perspectives. Fertil Steril 2017;108(3):407–15.e11.
6. Goldman RH, Kaser DJ, Missmer SA, et al. Fertility treatment for the transgender community: a public opinion study. J Assist Reprod Genet 2017;34(11):1457–67.
7. Ethics Committee of the American Society for Reproductive Medicine. Access to fertility services by transgender persons: an Ethics Committee opinion. Fertil Steril 2015;104(5):1111–5.
8. Committee on Health Care for Underserved Women. Committee opinion no. 512: health care for transgender individuals. Obstet Gynecol 2011;118(6):1454–8.
9. Tornello SL, Bos H. Parenting intentions among transgender individuals. LGBT health 2017;4(2):115–20.

10. Moore E, Wisniewski A, Dobs A. Endocrine treatment of transsexual people: a review of treatment regimens, outcomes, and adverse effects. J Clin Endocrinol Metab 2003;88(8):3467–73.
11. Matoso A, Khandakar B, Yuan S, et al. Spectrum of findings in orchiectomy specimens of persons undergoing gender confirmation surgery. Hum Pathol 2018;76: 91–9.
12. Leavy M, Trottmann M, Liedl B, et al. Effects of elevated beta-estradiol levels on the functional morphology of the testis - new insights. Sci Rep 2017;7:39931.
13. Schulze C. Response of the human testis to long-term estrogen treatment: morphology of sertoli cells, leydig cells and spermatogonial stem cells. Cell Tissue Res 1988;251(1):31–43.
14. Schneider F, Kliesch S, Schlatt S, et al. Andrology of male-to-female transsexuals: influence of cross-sex hormone therapy on testicular function. Andrology 2017; 5(5):873–80.
15. Lubbert H, Leo-Rossberg I, Hammerstein J. Effects of ethinyl estradiol on semen quality and various hormonal parameters in a eugonadal male. Fertil Steril 1992; 58(3):603–8.
16. Loverro G, Resta L, Dellino M, et al. Uterine and ovarian changes during testosterone administration in young female-to-male transsexuals. Taiwan J Obstet Gynecol 2016;55(5):686–91.
17. Unger CA. Hormone therapy for transgender patients. Transl Androl Urol 2016; 5(6):877–84.
18. Nakamura A, Watanabe M, Sugimoto M, et al. Dose-response analysis of testosterone replacement therapy in patients with female to male gender identity disorder. Endocr J 2013;60(3):275–81.
19. Caanen MR, Soleman RS, Kuijper EA, et al. Antimullerian hormone levels decrease in female-to-male transsexuals using testosterone as cross-sex therapy. Fertil Steril 2015;103(5):1340–5.
20. Ikeda K, Baba T, Noguchi H, et al. Excessive androgen exposure in female-to-male transsexual persons of reproductive age induces hyperplasia of the ovarian cortex and stroma but not polycystic ovary morphology. Hum Reprod 2013;28(2): 453–61.
21. De Roo C, Lierman S, Tilleman K, et al. Ovarian tissue cryopreservation in female-to-male transgender people: insights into ovarian histology and physiology after prolonged androgen treatment. Reprod Biomed Online 2017;34(6):557–66.
22. Perrone AM, Cerpolini S, Maria Salfi NC, et al. Effect of long-term testosterone administration on the endometrium of female-to-male (FtM) transsexuals. J Sex Med 2009;6(11):3193–200.
23. Practice Committees of American Society for Reproductive Medicine; Society for Assisted Reproductive Technology. Mature oocyte cryopreservation: a guideline. Fertil Steril 2013;99(1):37–43.
24. De Roo C, Tilleman K, T'Sjoen G, et al. Fertility options in transgender people. Int Rev Psychiatry 2016;28(1):112–9.
25. Kafetsoulis A, Brackett NL, Ibrahim E, et al. Current trends in the treatment of infertility in men with spinal cord injury. Fertil Steril 2006;86(4):781–9.
26. Van Voorhis BJ, Barnett M, Sparks AE, et al. Effect of the total motile sperm count on the efficacy and cost-effectiveness of intrauterine insemination and in vitro fertilization. Fertil Steril 2001;75(4):661–8.
27. Brannstrom M, Johannesson L, Bokstrom H, et al. Livebirth after uterus transplantation. Lancet 2015;385(9968):607–16.

28. Centers for Disease Control and Prevention ASfRM, Society for Assisted Reproductive Technology. 2015 Assisted reproductive technology national summary report. Atlanta (GA): Services UDoHaH; 2017.

29. Doyle JO, Richter KS, Lim J, et al. Successful elective and medically indicated oocyte vitrification and warming for autologous in vitro fertilization, with predicted birth probabilities for fertility preservation according to number of cryopreserved oocytes and age at retrieval. Fertil Steril 2016;105(2):459–66.e2.

30. Wallace SA, Blough KL, Kondapalli LA. Fertility preservation in the transgender patient: expanding oncofertility care beyond cancer. Gynecol Endocrinol 2014; 30(12):868–71.

31. Maxwell S, Noyes N, Keefe D, et al. Pregnancy outcomes after fertility preservation in transgender men. Obstet Gynecol 2017;129(6):1031–4.

32. Mitu K. Transgender reproductive choice and fertility preservation. AMA J Ethics 2016;18(11):1119–25.

33. Rodriguez-Wallberg KA, Dhejne C, Stefenson M, et al. Preserving eggs for men's fertility. a pilot experience with fertility preservation for female-to-male transsexuals in sweden. Fertil Steril 2014;102(3):e160–1.

34. Oktay K, Hourvitz A, Sahin G, et al. Letrozole reduces estrogen and gonadotropin exposure in women with breast cancer undergoing ovarian stimulation before chemotherapy. J Clin Endocrinol Metab 2006;91(10):3885–90.

35. Armuand G, Dhejne C, Olofsson JI, et al. Transgender men's experiences of fertility preservation: a qualitative study. Hum Reprod 2017;32(2):383–90.

36. Rowlands S, Amy JJ. Preserving the reproductive potential of transgender and intersex people. Eur J contracept Reprod Health Care 2018;23(1):58–63.

37. Light AD, Obedin-Maliver J, Sevelius JM, et al. Transgender men who experienced pregnancy after female-to-male gender transitioning. Obstet Gynecol 2014;124(6):1120–7.

38. Obedin-Maliver J, Makadon HJ. Transgender men and pregnancy. Obstet Med 2016;9(1):4–8.

39. Nahata L, Tishelman AC, Caltabellotta NM, et al. Low fertility preservation utilization among transgender youth. J Adolesc Health 2017;61(1):40–4.

40. Chen D, Simons L, Johnson EK, et al. Fertility preservation for transgender adolescents. J Adolesc Health 2017;61(1):120–3.

41. Linde R, Doelle GC, Alexander N, et al. Reversible inhibition of testicular steroidogenesis and spermatogenesis by a potent gonadotropin-releasing hormone agonist in normal men: an approach toward the development of a male contraceptive. N Engl J Med 1981;305(12):663–7.

42. Nielsen CT, Skakkebaek NE, Richardson DW, et al. Onset of the release of spermatozoa (spermarche) in boys in relation to age, testicular growth, pubic hair, and height. J Clin Endocrinol Metab 1986;62(3):532–5.

43. Hagenas I, Jorgensen N, Rechnitzer C, et al. Clinical and biochemical correlates of successful semen collection for cryopreservation from 12-18-year-old patients: a single-center study of 86 adolescents. Hum Reprod 2010;25(8):2031–8.

44. Haddad N, Al-Rabeeah K, Onerheim R, et al. Is ex vivo microdissection testicular sperm extraction indicated for infertile men undergoing radical orchiectomy for testicular cancer? Case report and literature review. Fertil Steril 2014;101(4): 956–9.

45. Picton HM, Wyns C, Anderson RA, et al. A European perspective on testicular tissue cryopreservation for fertility preservation in prepubertal and adolescent boys. Hum Reprod 2015;30(11):2463–75.

46. Stukenborg JB, Alves-Lopes JP, Kurek M, et al. Spermatogonial quantity in human prepubertal testicular tissue collected for fertility preservation prior to potentially sterilizing therapy. Hum Reprod 2018;33(9):1677–83.
47. Practice Committee of American Society for Reproductive Medicine. Ovarian tissue cryopreservation: a committee opinion. Fertil Steril 2014;101(5):1237–43.
48. Dittrich R, Hackl J, Lotz L, et al. Pregnancies and live births after 20 transplantations of cryopreserved ovarian tissue in a single center. Fertil Steril 2015;103(2): 462–8.
49. Donnez J, Silber S, Andersen CY, et al. Children born after autotransplantation of cryopreserved ovarian tissue. a review of 13 live births. Ann Med 2011;43(6): 437–50.
50. Van der Ven H, Liebenthron J, Beckmann M, et al. Ninety-five orthotopic transplantations in 74 women of ovarian tissue after cytotoxic treatment in a fertility preservation network: tissue activity, pregnancy and delivery rates. Hum Reprod 2016;31(9):2031–41.
51. Demeestere I, Simon P, Dedeken L, et al. Live birth after autograft of ovarian tissue cryopreserved during childhood. Hum Reprod 2015;30(9):2107–9.
52. Uzelac PS, Delaney AA, Christensen GL, et al. Live birth following in vitro maturation of oocytes retrieved from extracorporeal ovarian tissue aspiration and embryo cryopreservation for 5 years. Fertil Steril 2015;104(5):1258–60.

Gender Confirmation Surgery for the Endocrinologist

Sasha K. Narayan, BA[a], Tessalyn Morrison, BA[a],
Daniel D. Dugi III, MD[b], Scott Mosser, MD[c,1], Jens U. Berli, MD[d,*]

KEYWORDS

- Surgery • Gender confirmation • Transgender • Sex-reassignment • Mastectomy
- Phalloplasty • Vaginoplasty • Metoidioplasty

KEY POINTS

- Endocrinologists are key allies along a patient's journey through surgical transition.
- Facial gender confirmation surgery is a vital aspect of transition that augments or resects to alter misgendered features.
- Chest surgery (top surgery) does not require preoperative cessation of hormones. Trans-females benefit significantly from prior estrogen use to grow the breast, but augmentation is usually still required.
- Genital surgery (bottom surgery) may require preoperative estrogen cessation for venous thromboembolism risk. Testosterone does not seem to convey the same preoperative risk.
- Special consideration should be used in adolescent hormonal management because pubertal suppression will affect future surgical options.

Cross-sex hormones are a vital component of a patient's gender transition, but can fall short to completely align gender identity with the ideal phenotype. Gender confirmation surgery (GCS) provides an immediate, obvious change that helps to approximate the internal gender to the external appearance.

The World Professional Association for Transgender Health identifies GCS as medically necessary and therapeutic in the treatment of gender dysphoria to improve

Disclosure Statement: Dr S. Mosser holds stock options and shares for Remedly (EMR platform). Dr J.U. Berli has an Investigator Initiated Trial research grant through Allergan, Ireland. Drs S.K. Narayan, T. Morrison, and D.D. Dugi have nothing to disclose.
[a] School of Medicine, Oregon Health & Science University, 3181 Southwest Sam Jackson Park Road, Mail Code: L352A, Portland, OR 97239, USA; [b] Department of Urology, Oregon Health & Science University, 3303 Southwest Bond Avenue, Mail Code: CH10U, Portland, OR 97239, USA; [c] Saint Francis Memorial Hospital, San Francisco, CA, USA; [d] Department of Surgery, Division of Plastic and Reconstructive Surgery, Oregon Health & Science University, 3181 Southwest Sam Jackson Park Road, Mail Code: L352A, Portland, OR 97239, USA
[1] Present address: 450 Sutter Street #1000, San Francisco, CA 94108.
* Corresponding author.
E-mail address: berli@ohsu.edu

general well-being and sexual function.[1] A prospective study of 325 adults and adolescents in the Netherlands who underwent GCS in addition to hormonal therapy showed improvements in mean gender dysphoria scores (using the Utrecht Gender Dysphoria Score), body dissatisfaction, and psychological function,[2] which are results that agree with other retrospective analyses.[3–7]

Endocrinologists and mental health professionals are usually the first point of contact for patients seeking transition and are instrumental in guiding the patient through their journey. This article covers the basics of GCS and is intended to help nonsurgical providers guide their patients through surgical transition.

PREPARING FOR SURGERY

When talking to patients, it is helpful to point out that most surgical procedures devascularize the tissue. In preparing for surgery, all forms of nicotine should be stopped because they can impede wound healing and tissue survival. For this reason, other stimulants such as cocaine, methamphetamine, and even anorectics such as phentermine should also be stopped before surgery. For patients with dependency, documented abstinence is advocated. A urine test may be required by insurance carriers and/or surgeons before surgery.

Estrogen is stopped ideally 2 to 4 weeks before surgery to decrease the risk of thromboembolism; however, this is step controversial owing to the severe mental side effects some patients report and the low incidence of thromboembolism. Most surgeons agree that it should be discontinued before female bottom surgery owing to the extensive nature of the surgery and the need for postoperative bedrest.[8] In contrast, there is not enough evidence to suggest that testosterone cessation is associated with a lower risk of venous thromboembolism,[9] so many surgeons permit patients to continue testosterone before surgery. Calculation of the Caprini score can further assist in identifying high-risk patients who may benefit from perioperative venous thromboembolism prophylaxis.[10]

In patients with diabetes, the ideal hemoglobin A1c level is 7.0% or less before surgery.[11] Diabetic patients with preoperative hyperglycemia have been reported to have an increased risk of infection and cardiovascular morbidity in the perioperative period.[12]

GENDER CONFIRMATION PROCEDURES
Facial Gender Confirmation Surgery

Aligning the facial features with both gender identity and expression is one of the most important affirming interventions. It is vital for improved quality of life in all emotional, physical, and social domains.[13]

We like to think of the face as a gender mosaic, composed of both feminine and masculine features (**Fig. 1**). It is affirming to point out the already aligned facial features during consultation with the patient. Surgical treatment of the face to alter the areas of concern must address both the soft tissue and structural components. **Table 1** gives an overview of the most frequently performed surgeries and treatments.

Although the soft tissues may undergo changes owing to exogenous estrogen, hair follicles remain and definitive treatment requires electrolysis or laser hair removal. Laser resurfacing and chemical peels can assist in softening the skin appearance. Surgical rejuvenation procedures such as a face/neck lift or eyelid surgery are valuable adjuncts once the structural aspects, such as cheekbone and jawline, have been addressed.

The forehead is reduced by means of burring and/or bone resection. Frequently, the frontal sinus needs to be opened to allow for more aggressive reduction while preserving the bone covering the sinus. At the end of the surgery, the bone is therefore

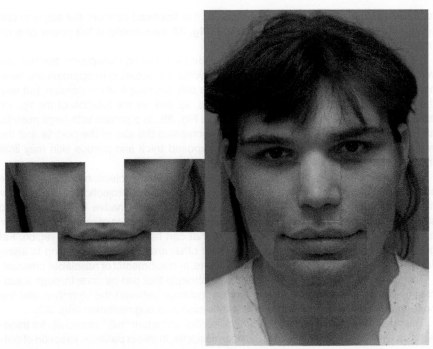

Fig. 1. Facial gender mosaic. This individual's cheek and perioral region are distinctly femi-nine, whereas the other aspects of her face have been masculinized through pubertal testosterone exposure.

Table 1 Overview of soft tissue and structural facial procedures		
Structural Procedure	**Associated Soft Tissue Procedure**	**Can Be Combined in One Surgery[a]**
Frontal bone reduction with or without frontal sinus setback	Brow lift	Yes
	Hairline advancement	Yes
	Hair transplantation	Yes
	Upper eyelid blepharoplasty	No
Rhinoplasty	With or without reduction of the skin envelope	Yes
		Yes
	Lip lift	
Cheek bone augmentation	Midfacial fat grafting	Yes but often either/or
	Lower eyelid blepharoplasty	Depends
Zygomatic arch reduction	Temporal fat grafting	Yes
Jawline shaping	Face lift/neck lift	No
	Masseter resection	Yes
Chin reduction and/or advancement (alternative chin implants)	Face lift/neck lift	No
Adams apple reduction	Neck lift, neck liposuction	Yes

[a] Author's opinion.

replaced and secured (**Fig. 2**). When closing the forehead incision, the surgeon can elevate the brow and advance the hairline. **Fig. 3**A demonstrates the power of such upper face procedures.

The nose makes up the central aspect of the face. During rhinoplasty, the skin envelope and cartilaginous and osseous frameworks are adjusted to approximate feminine proportions. Such alterations change not only the shape of the dorsum, but also the length, width, and projection of the nose, as well as the rotation of the tip. An example of femininizing rhinoplasty is seen in **Fig. 3**B. In a patient with large nostrils, an alar base wedge excision can assist in decreasing the size of the nostrils and the width of the nose. However, testosterone-exposed thick and porous skin may limit the result despite excision of excess skin.

The feminine midface ideal has high cheekbones with projection beyond the eye socket. Individual bony anatomy and aging may affect this projection, and a popular method of augmentation includes cheek implants. An alternative to implant-based structural cheek augmentation is autologous fat grafting. A midface lift in a patient affected more by aging is another modality that can help to feminize this region. Fat grafting is also a valuable adjunct to augment other areas of deflation owing to aging (ie, temporal hollowing, midfacial compartments, and submental or nasolabial creases).

The upper lip lift is a powerful feminizing technique that can be done through a subnasal incision. Not only does it shorten the distance between the vermillion and the nose, but this lift also provides upper lip eversion and augmentation (**Fig. 3**C).

The masculine lower face and neck can feel like an instant "tell," especially for transfemales with a prominent jaw, chin, or Adam's apple. In select patients, injection of botulinum toxin into the masseter muscles can achieve some decrease in facial width. Most patients, however, will require a reduction of the vertical height of the jawline as well as a resection of everted gonial angles and prominent masseter muscle through an intraoral incision. The chin can be reduced and/or advanced through the same

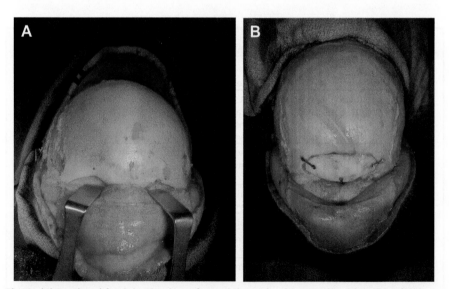

Fig. 2. (*A*) Forehead feminization is performed through a bicoronal incision that allows access to most of the frontal bone and periorbital region. (*B*) The anterior table of the frontal sinus is secured at the end of the procedure by means of rigid fixation. (*Courtesy of* Jens Berli, MD, Portland, Oregon.)

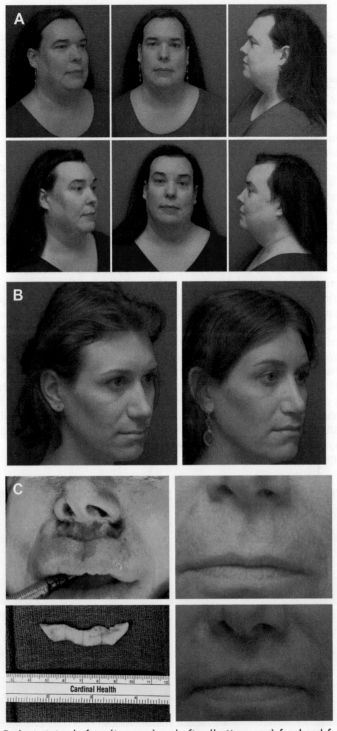

Fig. 3. (*A*) Patient status before (*top row*) and after (*bottom row*) forehead feminization with sinus set back and browlift. (*B*) Patient before (*left*) and after (*right*) forehead feminization (without sinus set back), rhinoplasty, and lip lift. (*C*) Patient status after lip lift (*bottom right*). (*Courtesy of* Jens Berli, MD, Portland, Oregon.)

incision. The Adam's apple is reduced through a small neck incision. Especially in older transfemale patients, a face and neck lift can assist in making the bony changes visible.

Chest Surgery

Colloquially, procedures for both masculinization and feminization of the chest are often referred to as top surgery.

Chest feminization

Many transfemales use the nonsurgical method of breast augmentation with removable prostheses placed in a brassiere. Although this technique can assist in social transition, it often does not treat gender dysphoria adequately. Exogenous estrogen (17-beta-estradiol) starts to encourage breast growth and body fat redistribution within 3 to 6 months, with full effects in 2 to 3 years and 2 to 5 years, respectively. Therefore, the World Professional Association for Transgender Health Standards of Care 7 recommend that patients undergo 12 months of hormone therapy before undergoing breast augmentation.[1] Estrogen's effect on glandular breast development is permanent, whereas its effect on body fat redistribution is reversible.[14]

Chest feminization addresses both the volume and shape of breast tissue. There are 2 broad categories: implant-based augmentation and fat injections. Fat grafting for breast augmentation is either done to further conceal an implant, craft realistic cleavage, or, infrequently, as the sole augmentation technique.[15] It is not recommended to use injections of medical grade silicone for augmentation.

The androgen-derived chest, even after being exposed to exogenous estrogen, differs from the natively estrogen-derived chest in key ways: there is not only less prominent breast tissue and an underdeveloped shape, but also incongruous chest width and breast proportionality. Endomorph patients with a higher body mass index and a wider chest (**Fig. 4**) require implants of considerable size and appropriate width or, if fat grafting, serial surgeries to reach the desired shape. When choosing implants, surgeons typically discuss 4 factors: type of implant, location, incision, and size. **Table 2** outlines an overview of choices.

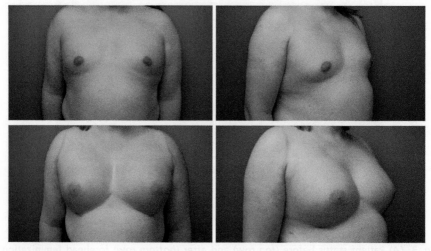

Fig. 4. The androgen-derived chest frequently presents with a wider breast base width and higher body mass index. This patient underwent subcutaneous augmentation using a 685-mL implant. (*Courtesy of* Jens Berli, MD, Portland, Oregon.)

Table 2 Options for breast implants and surgical approach	Options
Implant types	Silicone[a]
	Textured
	Round
	Shaped (tear drop)
	Smooth round
	Saline
Location	Submuscular
	Subglandular
	Subfascial
Incision	Inframammary
	Periareolar
	Axillary
	Umbilical (rare)
Size	~200–800 mL

[a] Colloquially, the term "Gummy Bear implant" refers to implants with a high cohesiveness/cross-linking of the silicone molecules leading to a more form-stable implant. These implants are often tear-drop shaped.

Postoperative care involves good brasserie support and early massage of the implant to soften the skin envelope and prevent capsular contracture. Most recently, textured implants have been associated with rare cases of anaplastic large cell lymphoma and should be used carefully.[16] This entity presents as a late-onset seroma and requires urgent referral to plastic surgery for removal of both implant and capsule, with cytology.

Chest masculinization

Before undergoing chest masculinization procedures, transmales or nonbinary individuals often achieve outcomes with chest binding at the price of rashes, chronic rib pain, and restrictive breathing problems. The preoperative evaluation should include a discussion of goals, including the importance of nipple sensation. Depending on the amount of breast tissue, elasticity, and amount of skin, the patient has various surgical options. The Fischer grading system (**Table 3**) can assist in determining which surgical techniques are associated with lower rates of aesthetic revisions.[17] Colloquially, there are 4 procedures that the transgender community will refer to and with which providers should be familiar.

Table 4 outlines the pros and cons for each of the 4 main procedures:

1. Keyhole,
2. Periareolar (circumareolar),
3. Inverted T/buttonhole, and
4. Double-incision with or without nipple graft.

Many patients only qualify for a double-incision procedure because it removes substantial breast tissue and addresses the ptosis and skin laxity that is created by chronic breast binding.[17] See **Fig. 5**A for an example of the results of the keyhole procedure and **Fig. 5**B for an example of the double incision with free nipple grafts result. Some patients, usually nonbinary identified, may opt to forego nipple grafting.[18] If they later desire nipples, 3-dimensional tattooing provides excellent aesthetic results.

Testosterone hormone therapy is not a prerequisite for mastectomy. However, many transmales have elected to use testosterone before surgery as an early part of their transition. The use of depo-testosterone over years in an individual with natively estrogen-derived breasts has been shown to induce histologic atrophy and fibrosis of the glandular breast tissue.[19] Testosterone has also been shown, at least in primates, to inhibit growth and have apoptotic effects in some breast cancer cell lines[20] Unlike cancer-related mastectomies, in chest masculinization, some breast tissue may be left behind. Although the risk of breast cancer is likely significantly decreased, we do not yet have enough evidence. Therefore, patients remain at some risk for breast cancer after surgery and should attend recommended screenings,[21] knowing that mammography is technically infeasible. For patients whose risk is increased (hereditary or genetic risk), other options such as MRI may be appropriate for new concerns.[22]

Table 3
Fischer grading system

Fischer Grade	Recommended Surgical Approach	Preop Anterior View	Preop Oblique View
1	Keyhole Peri/circumareolar		Grade 1
2A	Peri/circumareolar Extended circumareolar Double incision with or without free nipple grafts (if nipple-areola complex is at an unfavorable position)		Grade 2A
2B	Extended circumareolar Double incision with or without free nipple grafts		Grade 2B
3	Double incision with or without free nipple grafts T-anchor		Grade 3
4	Double incision with or without free nipple grafts		Grade 4

From Bluebond-Langner R, Berli JU, Sabino J, et al. Top surgery in transgender men: how far can you push the envelope? 2017;139:879; with permission.

Table 4
Overview and decision factors for various mastectomy approaches

Mastectomy Approach	Before and After Representations (Blue Lines Indicate Incisions)	Pros	Cons
Keyhole		Good for very small breasts. Most minimal scars, best chance of passing with long-term appearance.	Technically challenging, slightly higher incidence of contour irregularity.
Circumareolar (aka periareolar)	See attached image 4B	Used for minimal to mild skin laxity, natural scar placement around areolas.	May result in 'pleating' of skin around areolas. Limitations in quantity of skin removal exist, revision rate is higher, areolas can widen after surgery

(continued on next page)

Table 4
(continued)

Mastectomy Approach	Before and After Representations (Blue Lines Indicate Incisions)	Pros	Cons
Buttonhole/ T-anchor	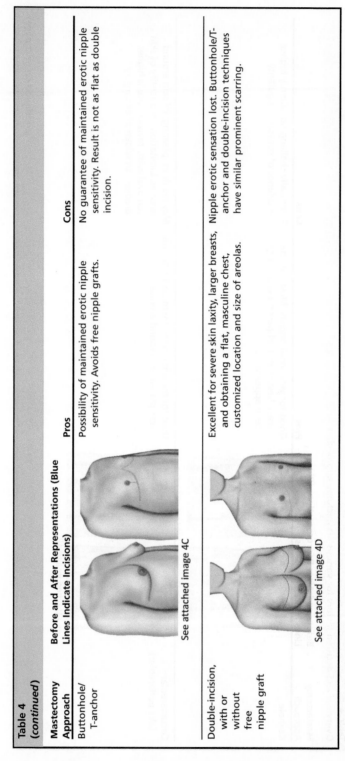 See attached image 4C	Possibility of maintained erotic nipple sensitivity. Avoids free nipple grafts.	No guarantee of maintained erotic nipple sensitivity. Result is not as flat as double incision.
Double-incision, with or without free nipple graft	See attached image 4D	Excellent for severe skin laxity, larger breasts, and obtaining a flat, masculine chest, customized location and size of areolas.	Nipple erotic sensation lost. Buttonhole/T-anchor and double-incision techniques have similar prominent scarring.

Courtesy of Dr Scott Mosser, MD, FACS, San Francisco, California.

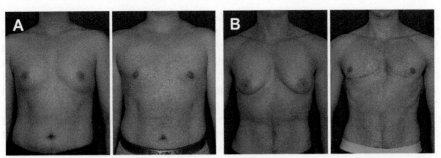

Fig. 5. (*A*) Patient before and after keyhole type chest masculinization. (*B*) Patient before and after double-incision and free nipple graft. (*Courtesy of* Scott Mosser, MD, San Francisco, California.)

Genital (Bottom) Surgery

Feminizing bottom surgery
Orchiectomy Some people pursue bilateral orchiectomy (removal of the testes) as their only genital surgery. This may relieve their dysphoria, and the removal of the testes can simplify their hormonal management without the need for androgen blockade. Typically, no scrotal skin is removed unless specifically requested, because patients are advised that scrotal skin is important if they later wish to undergo vaginoplasty.

Vaginoplasty Vaginoplasty describes a surgery to create a vaginal canal and the external female genitalia (vulva), including the clitoris, labia majora and minora, and the female urethral position (**Fig. 6**). The vaginal canal is created between the rectum, the bladder, and the urethra by dissecting through the pelvic floor muscles. The vaginal canal may be lined with genital skin flaps or skin grafts or, less commonly, a segment of ileum or sigmoid colon. When skin is used to line the neovaginal canal, that skin must be treated with laser hair removal or electrolysis before surgery to avoid bothersome hair growth within the neovagina.

Because the penile skin has a different blood supply from the glans and the deep structures of the penis, the skin can be separated and used to line the inner vulva

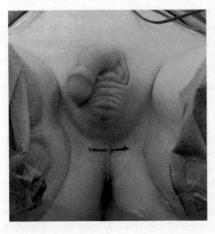
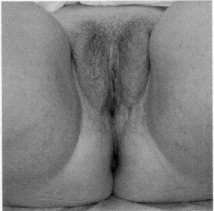

Fig. 6. Patient before and after feminizing vaginoplasty. (*Courtesy of* Daniel Dugi, MD, Portland, Oregon.)

and part of the neovaginal canal. The erectile tissue of the corpora of the penis and the testes are removed. The glans penis and its neurovascular bundle are decreased in size to form an erogenously sensate neoclitoris. Scrotal skin is used to create labia majora. Depending on the technique, penile skin or urethral tissue can be used to create the inner labia and a clitoral hood, one of the more challenging aspects of this surgery from an aesthetic standpoint. Patient satisfaction rates are high and most patients are able to achieve orgasm after surgery.[23]

Because of the natural process of wound contraction and because the neovagina passes through a newly created space in the pelvic floor muscles, patients must perform daily dilation of the neovagina with increasingly larger dilators to prevent stenosis and to maintain the depth and width of the vagina created at the time of surgery. The frequency of dilation decreases over the first year after surgery, but patients should expect to dilate, at least occasionally, life-long.

Vulvoplasty Vulvoplasty refers to surgery to create the external female genitalia, or vulva. This procedure is a part of vaginoplasty but, when used alone, vulvoplasty refers to surgery without the creation of a vaginal canal and supplants less accurate terms such as zero-depth vaginoplasty or cosmetic vaginoplasty. This procedure may be done for patients who prefer this configuration because they do not want to have receptive intercourse or upon surgeon recommendation owing to prior radical prostatectomy or pelvic radiation that would make dissection of the vaginal canal dangerous.[24] No preoperative permanent hair removal is necessary.

Masculinizing bottom surgery

Nonsurgical penile prostheses used in the underwear is often referred to as packing and is used frequently in social transition. For those people who desire a reconstructive autologous solution, the options for masculinizing bottom surgeries include metoidioplasty or phalloplasty. With either option, the individual's desire to urinate from the reconstructed glans guides the consultation. If so, the urethra needs to be lengthened through a phallus. If not, the urethra remains at the current anatomic location and options include a simple metoidioplasty or shaft-only phalloplasty. In these last cases, vaginectomy and hysterectomy are optional. If the patient chooses to urinate from the tip, there is increasing evidence to support the need for a vaginectomy at the time of urethral lengthening to assist in well-vascularized coverage of the reconstruction.[25]

Irrespective of a surgeon's methods, it is helpful to think of masculinizing bottom surgery as a modular set of surgical procedures where different available surgeries can be combined and staged in various ways. This complex and customized approach makes these procedures difficult to discuss in online forums or with nonsurgical providers. Even surgical providers are often not familiar with the procedure staging or surgical timelines of other surgeons. This article, therefore, cannot be considered comprehensive, although it attempts to provide a basic overview of the principles of masculinizing bottom surgical procedures.

Metoidioplasty Metoidioplasty (Greek: *forming toward male*) is a masculinizing genital surgery (**Fig. 7**) that uses the fact that the clitoris, the embryonic analog of the penis, grows in response to testosterone.[26] From an endocrinologic standpoint, a metoidioplasty is only possible if testosterone has had enough of an effect to lead to considerable clitoral growth because the lengthening of the unaffected clitoris would have little benefit. External pumps and dihydrotestosterone gel are adjunct methods frequently used by patients; however, there is little evidence to support any long-term benefit to length or girth. Patients with significant truncal fat will similarly not benefit as much from this procedure because the reconstruction may not be visible from above or allow

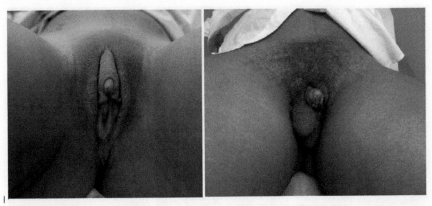

Fig. 7. Patient before and after metoidioplasty. (*Courtesy of* Daniel Dugi, MD, Portland, Oregon.)

for standing micturition. Although metoidioplasty preserves erogenous sensation, it generally does not allow for penetrative intercourse and, only in some cases, will it allow for standing urination. It is unknown exactly how many patients convert to a phalloplasty at a later stage, but it is certainly not insignificant in these authors' opinion. Some surgeons will do a metoidioplasty as a first stage procedure of a phalloplasty. The surgical steps include the release of the suspensory ligament that attaches to the pubic bone and urethral plate between the glans and external urethral meatus, thereby revealing the shaft. Tissue from the vulvar vestibule is used to create a lengthened urethra and shaft skin. Vaginectomy and testicular implants are also options in metoidioplasty.

Phalloplasty The principle of using analogous locoregional tissue is insufficient for the creation of a shaft and penile urethra that allow for consistent standing micturition and enough length for sexual intercourse. To perform the phalloplasty, transplanted tissue that comes with a blood supply (a flap) is used. This tissue can be transferred either as a random pattern flap (abdominal-based phalloplasty), a pedicled flap (thigh-based phalloplasty), or a free flap (from the radial forearm or back). Some surgeons use grafts to assist in urethral formation (ie, buccal graft). Similarly, skin grafts are used to cover donor defects (**Fig. 8**) and assist in the creation of the glans.

   Table 5 outlines the various options available to patients depending on their anatomy and goals. Although there are many possible options, most patients only qualify for a radial forearm phalloplasty (**Fig. 9**A) if they desire urethral lengthening owing to the thinness and pliability of the tissue. Very thin patients may prefer an anterolateral thigh free flap phalloplasty (**Fig. 9**B), although additional imaging may be needed to assess their anatomy because such phalloplasties are at risk of excessive girth. In creating a phallus from a shaft, the glansplasty is performed either at the time of tubularization of tissue, or as a subsequent procedure. See **Fig. 10** for a postoperative picture of a second-stage glansplasty.

   Although the benefits of, and how best to schedule, staging the phalloplasty are subject to ongoing debate, an overview of current options are found in **Table 6**. As mentioned elsewhere in this article, hysterectomy is a prerequisite when urethral lengthening is part of the surgical plan. Thus, fertility considerations are vital, especially in pediatric and young adult transgender patients.

   Patients who desire penetrative intercourse with their phallus will likely request an erectile implant. There are 2 broad categories of erectile implant: inflatable and

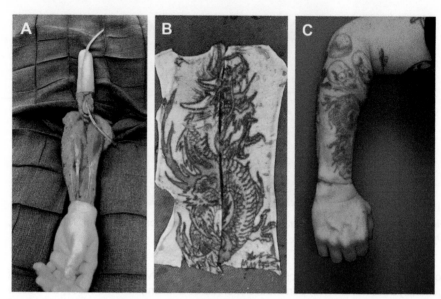

Fig. 8. (*A*) Radial forearm free flap phalloplasty donor site. (*B*) Harvested skin graft from thigh, including tattoo. (*C*) Healed forearm after reconstruction. (*Courtesy of* Jens Berli, MD, Portland, Oregon.)

Table 5
Components of various surgical masculinizing genital procedures

	Metoidioplasty, Simple	Metoidioplasty, Complete	Shaft Only	Tube within a Tube Phalloplasty or Composite Phalloplasty
Donor sites	Locoregional tissue	Locoregional tissue	ALT, RFFFP, abdominal, SCIP, TdAP	RFFFP, ALT, Fibula
Penile shaft	−	−	+	+
Penile urethra	−	−	−	+
Scrotoplasty	+/−	+	+/−	+
Urethral lengthening	−	+	1. None 2. To base 3. Perineal urostomy	+
Glansplasty	−	−	+	+
Erectile implant	−	−	+	+
Vaginectomy	+/−	+	+/−	+
Nerve connection	−	−	+	+
Hysterectomy	+/−	+	+/−	+

Abbreviations: −, not available/performed in that surgical option; +, present in that surgical option; +/−, may or may not be included in that surgical option; ALT, anterolateral thigh free flap; RFFFP, radial forearm free flap phalloplasty; SCIP, superficial circumflex iliac artery perforator (groin) flap; TdAP, thoracodorsal artery perforator flap.

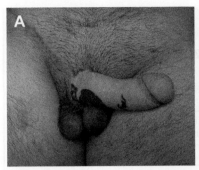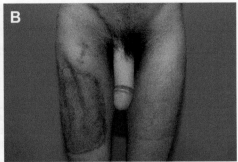

Fig. 9. (A) Healed radial forearm free flap phalloplasty. (B) Healed anterolateral thigh flap phalloplasty. (*Courtesy of* Jens Berli, MD, San Francisco, California.)

semimalleable. The inflatable implant involves a reservoir behind the pubic bone that directs fluid to fill a cylinder inside the shaft when initiated by a scrotal pump. A release valve drains the water from the cylinder to the reservoir, restoring the flaccid state. The semimalleable implant is manually shaped into the desired position. Unfortunately, both types of implant are fraught with complications. Aside from infection and extrusion, malfunction is the most notable issue. Because the semimalleable implants are persistently erect, they represent a higher risk for extrusion. Both implants need to be secured to the pubic bone in an effort to stabilize and decrease risk for extrusion. Currently there is no transgender-specific implant that is approved by the US Food and Drug Administration that addresses these complications. Osseointegrated prosthesis have been described in the literature, but are not commonly used.[27]

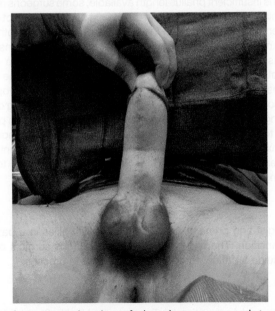

Fig. 10. Immediately postoperative view of glansplasty as a second-stage procedure on a well-healed radial forearm free flap phalloplasty. (*Courtesy of* Jens Berli, MD, Portland, Oregon.)

Table 6
An example of options for staging phalloplasty

Stage 1	Stage 2	Stage 3	Stage 4
Perineal masculinization[a] and creation of shaft and urethra			
Creation of neophallus with or without urethra	Perineal masculinization With or without glansplasty	Testicular implants With or without erectile implants	
Complete metoidioplasty	Creation of shaft and urethra and connection	Testicular implants With or without erectile implants	
Complete metoidioplasty	Creation of shaft and urethra	Delayed urethroplasty	Testicular implants With or without erectile implants

[a] Perineal masculinization: vaginectomy, urethral lengthening, scrotoplasty, and perineoplasty.

IMPORTANT CONSIDERATIONS FOR ADOLESCENTS

Surgical care of the adolescent is a field that has tremendous overlap with their endocrinologic care. Exogenous hormone substitution or blockade can significantly impact future surgical need. A transfemale who has had puberty blockers may not require any facial surgery to be affirmed in her gender. However, she will have less penile and scrotal tissue, necessitating additional skin harvest sites if she later desires penile-inversion vaginoplasty. If there is insufficient phallus length available, some surgeons may recommend a colonic vaginoplasty.[28] It is important that the patient be counseled not only on the benefits of these interventions, but also on the potential downsides and other options.

Adolescent transgender patients and their families need to be counseled sensitively on their thoughts surrounding their fertility and future reproductive goals. Many of these surgical options irreversibly impact their fertility by removing the gonads. Before these procedures are undertaken, sperm and oocytes may be cryopreserved. This step, however, comes with substantial costs. Another fertility-sparing option is to offer a unilateral salpingo-oophorectomy. This procedure leaves 1 ovary in place at the time of hysterectomy to preserve future fertility and allow for reserve hormones in the event of inaccessible exogenous androgens. For these reasons, adolescent patients especially are best treated at a multidisciplinary center with easy access to all associated services, including fertility preservation.

SUMMARY

The endocrinologist and primary care provider are key allies in a patient's pathway along gender transition. The understanding of the various surgical options enables the provider to guide a patient through this complicated process.

REFERENCES

1. World Professional Association for Transgender Health. Standards of care for the health of transsexual, transgender, and gender nonconforming people. WPATH; 2011. p. 54–109.

2. Smith YL, Van Goozen SH, Kuiper AJ, et al. Sex reassignment: outcomes and predictors of treatment for adolescent and adult transsexuals. Psychol Med 2005;35(1):89–99.
3. Green R, Fleming D. Transsexual surgery follow-up. Status in the 1990s. Annu Rev Sex Res 1990;1(1):163–74.
4. Eldh J, Berg A, Gustafsson M. Long-term follow-up after sex reassignment surgery. Scand J Plast Reconstr Surg Hand Surg 1997;31(1):39–45.
5. Pfäfflin F, Junge A. Sex reassignment: Thirty years of international follow-up studies after sex reassignment surgery: a comprehensive review, 1961–1991. Düsseldorf (Germany): Symposion; 2003.
6. Gijs L, Brewaeys A. Surgical treatment of gender dysphoria in adults and adolescents: recent developments, effectiveness, and challenges. Annu Rev Sex Res 2007;18:178–224.
7. Johansson A, Sundbom E, Höjerback T, et al. A five-year follow-up study of Swedish adults with gender identity disorder. Arch Sex Behav 2010;39(6):1429–37.
8. Hembree WC, Cohen-Kettenis PT, Gooren L, et al. Endocrine treatment of gender-dysphoric/gender-incongruent persons: an endocrine society clinical practice guideline. J Clin Endocrinol Metab 2017;102(11):3869–903.
9. Elamin MB, Garcia MZ, Murad MH, et al. Effect of sex steroid use on cardiovascular risk in transsexual individuals: a systematic review and meta-analyses. Clin Endocrinol (Oxf) 2010;72(1):1–10.
10. Gould MK, Garcia DA, Wren SM, et al. Prevention of VTE in nonorthopedic surgical patients: antithrombotic therapy and prevention of thrombosis, 9th ed: American College of Chest Physicians Evidence-Based Clinical Practice Guidelines. Chest 2012;141(2 Suppl):e227S–77S.
11. Underwood P, Askari R, Hurwitz S, et al. Preoperative A1C and clinical outcomes in patients with diabetes undergoing major noncardiac surgical procedures. Diabetes Care 2014;37(3):611–6.
12. Malone DL, Genuit T, Tracy JK, et al. Surgical site infections: reanalysis of risk factors. J Surg Res 2002;103(1):89.
13. Ainsworth TA, Spiegel JH. Quality of life of individuals with and without facial feminization surgery or gender reassignment surgery. Qual Life Res 2010;19(7):1019–24.
14. Wesp LM, Deutsch MB. Hormonal and surgical treatment options for transgender women and transfeminine spectrum persons. Psychiatr Clin North Am 2017;4:99–111.
15. Colebunder B, Brondeel S, D'Arpa S, et al. An update on the surgical treatment for transgender patients. Sex Med Rev 2017;5:103–9.
16. De Boer M, van der Sluis WB, de Boer JP, et al. Breast implant-associated anaplastic large-cell lymphoma in a transgender woman. Aesthet Surg J 2017;37(8):83–7.
17. Bluebond-Langner R, Berli JU, Sabino J, et al. Top surgery in transgender men: how far can you push the envelope? Plast Reconstr Surg 2017;139:873–83.
18. Esmonde N, Heston A, Ramly E, et al. What is "non-binary" and what do I need to know? A primer for surgeons providing chest surgery for transgender patients. Aesthet Surg J 2018. https://doi.org/10.1093/asj/sjy166.
19. Merkel KHH, Gross U. Histomorphology of the human female breast after long-term testosterone administration. Pathol Res Pract 1981;171(3):411–6.
20. Somboonporn W, Davis SR, National Health and Medical. Testosterone effects on the breast: implications for testosterone therapy for women. Endocr Rev 2004;25(3):374–88.

21. Pivo S, Montes J, Schwartz S, et al. Breast cancer risk assessment and screening in transgender patients. Clin Breast Cancer 2016;17(5):225–7.
22. Deutsch MB. Guidelines for the primary and gender-affirming care of transgender and gender nonbinary people. 2nd edition. San Francisco (CA): Center of Excellence for Transgender Health, Department of Family and Community Medicine, University of California; 2016.
23. Horbach SE, Bouman MB, Smit JM, et al. Outcome of vaginoplasty in male-to-female transgenders: a systematic review of surgical techniques. J Sex Med 2015;12(6):1499–512.
24. Jiang D, Witten J, Berli J, et al. Does depth matter? factors affecting choice of vulvoplasty over vaginoplasty as gender-affirming genital surgery for transgender women. J Sex Med 2018;15(6):902–6.
25. Massie JP, Morrison SD, Wilson SC, et al. Phalloplasty with urethral lengthening: addition of a vascularized bulbospongiosus flap from vaginectomy reduces postoperative urethral complications. Plast Reconstr Surg 2017;140(4):551e–8e.
26. Perovic SV, Djordjevic ML. Metoidioplasty: a variant of phalloplasty in female transsexuals. BJU Int 2003;92(9):981–5.
27. Selvaggi G, Branemark R, Elander A, et al. Titanium-bone-anchored penile epithesis: preoperative planning and immediate postoperative results. J Plast Surg Hand Surg 2015;49(1):40–4.
28. Salgado CJ, Nugent A, Kuhn J, et al. Primary sigmoid vaginoplasty in transwomen: technique and outcomes. Biomed Res Int 2018;2018:4907208.

Osteoporosis and Bone Health in Transgender Persons

Mary O. Stevenson, MD[a], Vin Tangpricha, MD, PhD[b,c,*,1]

KEYWORDS

- Osteoporosis • Bone density • Transgender • Hormone therapy
- Gender affirmation • Dual-energy x-ray absorptiometry

KEY POINTS

- Gender-affirming hormone therapy in transgender people has been shown to maintain or improve bone density with unknown effect on fracture risk.
- Screening for osteoporosis should be based on clinical risk factors, including time off sex steroid hormone therapy after gonadal removal.
- Children and adolescents may be at risk for decreasing bone density while on pubertal blockade without sex steroid hormone replacement.
- Transgender people with the highest fracture risk should receive osteoporosis therapy based on guidelines for the general population.

INTRODUCTION

Transgender children and adults receive gender-affirming hormone therapy to improve gender dysphoria and to better align their physical and emotional characteristics with their affirmed gender.[1] Gender-affirming hormone therapy includes the sex steroid hormones in transgender men and women and medications to lower testosterone such as spironolactone in transgender women.[2] Gonadotropin-releasing hormone (GnRH) agonists can also be used to delay puberty in youth and lowers

Funding sources: Supported by the National Center for Advancing Translational Sciences of the National Institutes of Health under Award Number UL1TR002378.

[a] Division of Endocrinology, Metabolism and Lipids, Department of Medicine, Emory University School of Medicine, 101 Woodruff Circle Northeast, WMRB 1028, Atlanta, GA 30322, USA;
[b] Division of Endocrinology, Metabolism and Lipids, Department of Medicine, Emory University School of Medicine, 101 Woodruff Circle Northeast, WRMB 1301, Atlanta, GA 30322, USA;
[c] Atlanta VA Medical Center, 1670 Clairmont Road Northeast, Decatur, GA 30300, USA
[1] Senior author.
* Corresponding author. Division of Endocrinology, Metabolism and Lipids, Department of Medicine, Emory University School of Medicine, 101 Woodruff Circle Northeast, WRMB 1301, Atlanta, GA 30322.
E-mail address: vin.tangpricha@emory.edu

testosterone in transgender women. Both these therapies can impact bone health, which has been a concern in transgender populations.

The most recent US population studies estimate that approximately 0.6% of adults, or 1.4 million Americans, identify as transgender.[3] There are no current estimates of the prevalence of osteoporosis or low bone mass in transgender individuals in the United States. Furthermore, there is a paucity of data regarding fracture rates in these patients.

Both sex steroids—estrogen and testosterone—have been shown to be important factors in bone formation during puberty and bone turnover during adulthood.[4] During puberty, males attain a larger, but not denser, bone mass than females owing to greater periosteal apposition from testosterone stimulation.[5] There is no difference in peak volumetric bone mineral density (BMD) or the amount of bone within the periosteal envelope (quantified by grams per cubic centimeter) between the sexes.[5] Estrogen plays an important role in the acquisition of healthy bone in males.[6] Males with inactivating mutations in the estrogen receptor and aromatase genes have low bone mass despite normal or high levels of testosterone.[7–9] Both men and women in hypogonadal states have higher rates of osteoporosis, and treatment with hormone supplementation has been shown to improve bone density.[10–14]

This review focuses on the clinical aspects of the screening and diagnosis of osteoporosis and the treatment of low bone mass in transgender males and females. Topics regarding bone mass in children and adolescents are also covered.

DIAGNOSIS AND SCREENING
Diagnosis of Osteoporosis in Trans Persons

There are no studies that have evaluated whether clinicians should use birth assigned sex or affirmed gender for the determination of the T-score or the Z-score. The T-score is a value calculated by comparing bone density in postmenopausal women or men over the age of 50 to the bone density of a healthy gender matched adult at the time of peak bone mass.[15] A T-score value of −2.5 or less is considered osteoporosis; a T-score between −1.0 and −2.5 is considered low bone mass (osteopenia).[15] The Z-score is used for patients under the age of 50 and is a value calculated by comparing an individual's bone density to age-, sex-, and ethnicity-matched controls.[15]

The International Society for Clinical Densitometry recommends use of a "Caucasian (non-race adjusted) female reference for cisgender men and women of all ethnic groups."[16] This recommendation is primarily based on the availability of fracture data by bone density measurement. Thus, using the Caucasian female reference range would better reflect fracture risk in both transgender women and men. Finally, the presence of fragility fractures or the occurrence of hip or vertebral fracture in the absence of major trauma independent of BMD would constitute a diagnosis of osteoporosis.[17]

Screening in Trans Women

The recommended screening modality for osteoporosis is dual energy x-ray absorptiometry of the lumbar spine, total hip, and femoral neck.[18] There are few studies that examine the prevalence of osteoporosis and low bone density in transgender women based on dual energy x-ray absorptiometry. A study from Belgium found that, in hormone treatment–naive transgender women, the prevalence of osteoporosis and low bone density in the lumbar spine was 16% and 32%, respectively (based on the male reference range).[19] The authors postulated that the high prevalence of osteoporosis and low bone density in young transgender women was due to a less active lifestyle as determined by a physical activity questionnaire.[19]

Hormone therapy is associated with increases in BMD in trans women. A recent metaanalysis demonstrated a statistically significant increase in BMD in transgender women at 12 and 24 months in the lumbar spine compared with baseline across 9 studies.[20] The clinical significance of this change in BMD on fracture risk is unknown; however, estrogen has been shown to increase bone density and decrease fracture risk in postmenopausal cisgender women.[21] There has been no observed difference in fracture rates between trans women compared with control men.[22,23]

The Endocrine Society Practice Guidelines[2] recommend that clinicians obtain BMD for screening purposes in trans women when risk factors for low bone density exist, such as smoking, low body weight, chronic corticosteroid use, heavy alcohol use,[24] and particularly in patients who stop hormone therapy after undergoing gonadectomy. Various risk factors to consider are presented in **Fig. 1**.

Screening in Trans Men

There are a handful of studies that provide data on bone density in transgender men before the start of hormone therapy. In 1 study, the bone density at lumbar, femoral neck and total hip (reported in grams per square centimeter) of 16 trans men compared with control women was similar.[25] In another study, a slightly higher bone density was seen in the femoral neck in trans men compared with control cisgender females (1.02 vs 0.95 g/cm^2, respectively; $P = .02$).[26]

During treatment, a recent metaanalysis found no statistically significant changes in BMD at 12 and 24 months after the initiation of treatment compared with baseline values in testosterone-treated trans men.[20] One study included in the metaanalysis did find a positive effect of testosterone treatment of bone density with an increase in mean BMD of 7.8% at the femoral neck over a 2-year period.[27] There are few

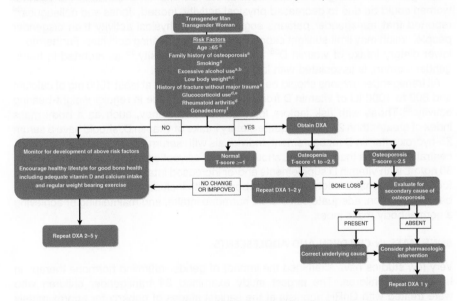

Fig. 1. Suggested approach to screening and the treatment of adult transgender patients. [a] American Association of Clinical Endocrinology/American College of Endocrinology Guidelines.[39] [b] Three or more drinks per day. [c] Weighing less than 127 lbs or a body mass index (BMI) of less than 20 kg/m. [d] Risk factors included in the FRAX tool[40]. [e] Prednisolone 5 mg/d or more for 3 months or more, current or past. [f] Endocrine Society Clinical Practice Guidelines.[2] [g] Bone loss greater than least significant change.

data regarding fracture rates in transgender men. In a 1-year prospective study, 53 trans men receiving testosterone therapy over a 1-year period had no observed osteoporotic fractures.[28] Adequate levels of testosterone therapy are needed to maintain bone density, and luteinizing hormone levels in the normal range have been shown to be a useful marker in determining sufficient levels of testosterone therapy to prevent bone loss (ie, an inverse relationship between BMD and serum luteinizing hormone levels).[29]

Screening for osteoporosis in trans men is appropriate in patients who stop or are intermittently compliant with testosterone therapy, especially in those who have undergone a gonadectomy.[2] In 1 study done in Singapore, postgonadectomy trans men both on regular testosterone treatment and those off testosterone treatment or intermittently compliant with treatment were found to have a lower BMD as compared with values in trans men without gonadectomy.[30] In concordance with the Endocrine Society Clinical Practice guidelines,[2] screening for osteoporosis is appropriate when risks for bone loss are present and potentially in those patients who have increased luteinizing hormone values. Other features to consider are presented in **Fig. 1**.

NONPHARMACOLOGIC THERAPY IN TRANSGENDER PERSONS FOR BONE HEALTH

Vitamin D, calcium, and weight-bearing activity should be encouraged for all transgender persons to ensure optimal bone health. Studies[19,31] examining vitamin D status in transgender adults have demonstrated mean serum 25-hydroxyvitamin D concentrations below the optimal level of 30 ng/mL (75 nmol/L) as suggested by the Endocrine Society[32] and American Association of Clinical Endocrinologists.[33] Van Caenegem and colleagues[19] reported that the low vitamin D status in transgender women could be due to decreased physical activity. Indeed, Jones and colleagues[34] reported that transgender persons engage in less physical activity than cisgender people, which may limit sunlight exposure and weight-bearing activities. Furthermore, lower dietary intake of vitamin D[35] and increased adiposity,[36] as reported in transgender women, is associated with lower vitamin D status.

All transgender persons should be encouraged to ingest at least 1000 mg of calcium and 800 to 1000 IU of vitamin D from the diet and engage in regular weight-bearing activity.[33] Those with risk factors for vitamin D deficiency, such as a body mass index of greater than 27 or inadequate dietary intake of vitamin D, should have a serum 25-hydroxyvitamin D measurement. Individuals with serum 25-hydroxyvitamin D concentrations of less than 30 ng/mL should attempt correction of the level to greater than 30 ng/mL with vitamin D supplements and/or increased intake of vitamin D–containing foods. Other considerations to improve bone health include limiting alcohol intake, tobacco cessation, adequate sex steroid hormone intake, and maintaining or achieving a normal body mass index.

BONE MASS IN CHILDREN AND ADOLESCENTS

Very few studies have examined the impact of gender-affirming hormone therapy in transgender children. The largest study examined 34 transgender children who were treated with GnRH agonists at the earliest stages of puberty for approximately 1 to 2 years followed by gender-affirming hormone therapy for 5 years.[37] They reported no change in absolute BMD (aBMD) of the spine in trans girls during GnRH therapy and slight increase in aBMD after the initiation of gender-affirming hormone therapy. In trans boys, the investigators reported significant decreases in aBMD of the spine at the start of GnRH therapy and stabilization of aBMD of the spine after the initiation of gender-affirming hormone therapy. However, in both groups of trans boys and trans girls, the Z-scores of the spine were less than 0. This small study raises concerns regarding prolonged GnRH therapy on bone health without sex steroid hormone replacement in transgender children and adults. Further studies should investigate the timing and duration of GnRH therapy that may impact bone health in postpubertal children and adults.

TREATMENT OF OSTEOPOROSIS IN TRANSGENDER PERSONS

Most of the studies that have been conducted in transgender populations have been of individuals under the age of 50. According to World Health Organization criteria, osteoporosis cannot be diagnosed using T-scores alone in individuals less than the age of 50.[38] There are no published reports examining the safety and efficacy of pharmacologic agents such as bisphosphonates in the treatment of osteoporosis in transgender populations. Therefore, in the absence of any transgender-specific data, pharmacologic therapy should be based on criteria put forth by guidelines by international societies in cisgender populations.[17]

SUMMARY

There has been a recent increasing interest in both the short- and long-term effects of sex steroid hormones on bone health in transgender persons. Based on the available data, hormone therapy seems to maintain or improve bone density in transgender adults in short-term follow-up. For transgender children and adolescents, there is concern that GnRH agonist use before the initiation of sex steroid hormones may put patients at risk for decreasing bone density. Both pharmacologic and nonpharmacologic treatments for transgender persons follow the same guidelines as in cisgender persons. See **Fig. 1** for a suggested approach to the screening and treatment of adult transgender patients.

More studies are needed to assess the long-term effects of hormone therapy on bone density and the clinical impact of these changes on fracture rates. As the population of transgender persons on hormone therapy ages, this consideration will become especially important. Further studies are also required to assess the timing and duration of GnRH agonists in transgender youth and the associated effects on bone density.

REFERENCES

1. Coleman E, Bockting W, Botzer M, et al. Standards of care for the health of transsexual, transgender, and gender-nonconforming people, version 7. Int J Transgend 2012;13:165–232.
2. Hembree WC, Cohen-Kettenis PT, Gooren L, et al. Endocrine treatment of gender-dysphoric/gender-incongruent persons: an endocrine society clinical practice guideline. J Clin Endocrinol Metab 2017;102(11):3869–903.
3. Flores AR, Herman JL, Gates GJ, et al. How many adults identify as transgender in the United States? Los Angeles: The Williams Institute; 2016.
4. Turner RT, Riggs BL, Spelsberg TC. Skeletal effects of estrogen. Endocr Rev 1994;15:275–300.
5. Seeman E. Sexual dimorphism in skeletal size, density, and strength. J Clin Endocrinol Metab 2001;89(10):4576–84.
6. Gennari L, Khosla S, Bilezikian JP. Estrogen and fracture risk in men. J Bone Miner Res 2008;23:1548–51.

7. Smith EP, Boyd J, Frank GR, et al. Estrogen resistance caused by a mutation in the estrogen receptor gene in a man. N Engl J Med 1994;331:1056–61.

8. Morishima A, Grumbach MM, Simpson ER, et al. Aromatase deficiency in male and female siblings caused by a novel mutation and the physiological role of estrogens. J Clin Endocrinol Metab 1995;80:3689–98.

9. Carani C, Qin K, Simoni M, et al. Effect of testosterone and estradiol in a man with aromatase deficiency. N Engl J Med 1997;337:91–5.

10. Behre HM, Kliesch S, Leifke E, et al. Long-term effect of testosterone therapy on bone mineral density in hypogonadal men. J Clin Endocrinol Metab 1997;82:2386.

11. Snyder PJ, Kopperdahl DL, Stephens-Shields AJ, et al. Effect of testosterone treatment on volumetric bone density and strength in older men with low testosterone: a controlled clinical trial. JAMA Intern Med 2017;177:471.

12. Finkelstein JS, Klibanski A, Neer RM, et al. Increases in bone density during treatment of men with idiopathic hypogonadotropic hypogonadism. J Clin Endocrinol Metab 1989;69:776.

13. Pacifici R. Estrogen, cytokines, and pathogenesis of postmenopausal osteoporosis. J Bone Miner Res 1996;11:1043–51.

14. Wells G, Tugwell P, Shea B, et al. Meta-analyses of therapies for postmenopausal osteoporosis. V. Meta-analysis of the efficacy of hormone replacement therapy in treating and preventing osteoporosis in postmenopausal women. Endocr Rev 2002;23(4):529–39.

15. International Society for Clinical Densitometry. 2013 official positions—adult. Available at: https://www.iscd.org/official-positions/2013-iscd-official-positions-adult/. Accessed March 13, 2018.

16. Shepherd JA, Schousboe JT, Broy SB, et al. Executive summary of the 2015 ISCD position development conference on advanced measures from DXA and QCT: fracture prediction beyond BMD. J Clin Densitom 2015;18(3):274–86.

17. Cosman F, de Beur SJ, LeBoff MS, et al. Clinician's guide to prevention and treatment of osteoporosis. Osteoporos Int 2014;25(10):2359–81.

18. World Health Organization. Assessment of fracture risk and its application to screening for postmenopausal osteoporosis: report of a WHO study group [meeting held in Rome from 22 to 25 June 1992]. Geneva: World Health Organization; 1994.

19. Van Caenegem E, Taes Y, Wierckx K, et al. Low bone mass is prevalent in male-to-female transsexual persons before the start of cross-sex hormonal therapy and gonadectomy. Bone 2013;54(1):92–7.

20. Singh-Ospina N, Maraka S, Rodriguez-Gutierrez R, et al. Effect of sex steroids on the bone health of transgender individuals: a systematic review and meta-analysis. J Clin Endocrinol Metab 2017;102(11):3904–13.

21. Jackson RD, Wactawski-Wende J, LaCroix AZ, et al. Women's Health Initiative Investigators: effects of conjugated equine estrogen on risk of fractures and BMD in postmenopausal women with hysterectomy: results from the women's health initiative randomized trial. J Bone Miner Res 2006;21:817–28.

22. Lapauw B, Taes Y, Simoens S, et al. Body composition, volumetric and areal bone parameters in male-to-female transsexual persons. Bone 2008;43:1016–21.

23. Sosa M, Jódar E, Arbelo E, et al. Bone mass, bone turnover, vitamin D, and estrogen receptor gene polymorphisms in male to female transsexuals: effects of estrogenic treatment on bone metabolism of the male. J Clin Densitom 2003;6:297–304.

24. World Health Organization. Prevention and management of osteoporosis: report of a WHO scientific group. Geneva: World Health Organization; 2003.
25. Van Caenegem E, Wierckx K, Taes Y, et al. Bone mass, bone geometry, and body composition in female-to-male transsexual persons after long-term cross-sex hormonal therapy. J Clin Endocrinol Metab 2012;97(7):2503–11.
26. Haraldsen IR, Haug E, Falch J, et al. Cross-sex pattern of bone mineral density in early onset gender identity disorder. Horm Behav 2007;52:334–43.
27. Turner A, Chen TC, Barber TW, et al. Testosterone increases bone mineral density in female-to-male transsexuals: a case series of 15 subjects. Clin Endocrinol (Oxf) 2004;61(5):560–6.
28. Wierckx K, Van Caenegem E, Schreiner T, et al. Cross-sex hormone therapy in trans persons is safe and effective at short-time follow-up: results from the European network for the investigation of gender incongruence. J Sex Med 2014;1: 1999–2011.
29. van Kesteren P, Lips P, Gooren LJ, et al. Long- term follow-up of bone mineral density and bone metabolism in transsexuals treated with cross-sex hormones. Clin Endocrinol (Oxf) 1998;48(3):347–54.
30. Goh HH, Ratnam SS. Effects of hormone deficiency, androgen therapy and calcium supplementation on bone mineral density in female transsexuals. Maturitas 1997;26:45–52.
31. Wiepjes CM, Vlot MC, Klaver M, et al. Bone mineral density increases in trans persons after 1 year of hormonal treatment: a multicenter prospective observational study. J Bone Miner Res 2017;32(6):1252–60.
32. Holick MF, Binkley NC, Bischoff-Ferrari HA, et al, Endocrine Society. Evaluation, treatment, and prevention of vitamin D deficiency: an Endocrine Society clinical practice guideline. J Clin Endocrinol Metab 2011;96(7):1911–30.
33. Hurley DL, Binkley N, Camacho PM, et al. The use of vitamins and minerals in skeletal health: American Association of Clinical Endocrinology (AACE/ACE) position statement. Endocr Pract 2018. https://doi.org/10.4158/PS-2018-0050.
34. Jones BA, Haycraft E, Bouman WP, et al. the levels and predictors of physical activity engagement within the treatment-seeking transgender population: a matched control study. J Phys Act Health 2018;15(2):99–107.
35. Vilas MVA, Rubalcava G, Becerra A, et al. Nutritional status and obesity prevalence in people with gender dysphoria. AIMS Public Health 2014;1(3):137–46.
36. Klaver M, de Blok CJM, Wiepjes CM, et al. Changes in regional body fat, lean body mass and body shape in trans persons using cross-sex hormonal therapy: results from a multicenter prospective study. Eur J Endocrinol 2018;178(2): 165–73.
37. Klink D, Caris M, Heijboer A, et al. Bone mass in young adulthood following gonadotropin-releasing hormone analog treatment and cross-sex hormone treatment in adolescents with gender dysphoria. J Clin Endocrinol Metab 2015;100(2): E270–5.
38. World Health Organization. Assessment of fracture risk and its application to screening for postmenopausal osteoporosis. World Health Organ Tech Rep Ser 1994;843:1–129.
39. Camacho PM, Petak SM, Binkley N, et al. American Association of Clinical Endocrinologists and American College of Endocrinology clinical practice guidelines for the diagnosis and treatment of postmenopausal osteoporosis - 2016. Endocr Pract 2016;22:1–42.
40. Kanis JA, Oden A, Johansson H, et al. FRAX and its applications to clinical practice. Bone 2009;44:734–43.

Dermatologic Conditions in Transgender Populations

Howa Yeung, MD[a,b,*], Benjamin Kahn, BA[a], Bao Chau Ly, BS[a],
Vin Tangpricha, MD, PhD[c,d]

KEYWORDS

- Transgender • Dermatology • Acne • Hair loss • Hirsutism • Keloid
- Gender affirmation

KEY POINTS

- Skin conditions often are underdiagnosed and undertreated in transgender patients despite potential for significant impairments in quality of life and mental health from skin diseases.
- Hormone therapy affects the skin and changes the prevalence and severity of many dermatologic conditions, including acne, male pattern hair loss, hirsutism, pseudofolliculitis barbae, and more.
- Clinicians caring for transgender persons should recognize and address common dermatologic conditions relevant to gender-affirming treatments.

INTRODUCTION

Transgender persons, in particular those receiving gender-affirming hormone and/or surgical treatments, may face specific dermatologic concerns. Hormone therapies and gender-affirming procedures can affect the skin and change the prevalence and presentation of routine skin conditions. Transgender patients with dermatologic disease may face body image dissatisfaction, which is closely tied to levels of gender dysphoria, anxiety, depression, and other secondary health problems.[1] Transgender patients also face greater barriers to care and often benefit from a comprehensive approach to care from providers they do see.[2] Therefore, it is important for clinicians caring for transgender persons to recognize and address common dermatologic

Disclosures: Dr H. Yeung received honorarium from Syneos (InVentiv) Health. The other authors have nothing to disclose.
[a] Department of Dermatology, Emory University School of Medicine, 1525 Clifton Road NE, Suite 100, Atlanta, GA 30322, USA; [b] Regional Telehealth Services, Veterans Integrated Service Network 7, 250 N Arcadia Avenue, Decatur, GA 30030, USA; [c] Division of Endocrinology, Metabolism and Lipids, Department of Medicine, Emory University School of Medicine, 101 Woodruff Circle Northeast, WRMB 1301, Atlanta, GA 30322, USA; [d] Atlanta VA Medical Center, 1670 Clairmont Road Northeast, Decatur, GA 30300, USA
* Corresponding author. Department of Dermatology, Emory University School of Medicine, 1525 Clifton Road NE, Suite 100, Atlanta, GA 30322.
E-mail address: howa.yeung@emory.edu

Endocrinol Metab Clin N Am 48 (2019) 429–440
https://doi.org/10.1016/j.ecl.2019.01.005
0889-8529/19/Published by Elsevier Inc.

endo.theclinics.com

conditions relevant to gender-affirming treatments This article reviews the clinical presentations, diagnosis, and treatment of skin conditions common in transgender patients, particularly for transmasculine and transfeminine patients undergoing gender-affirming endocrine or surgical therapies, as well as indications for dermatology referral.

HORMONE THERAPY

Gender-affirming hormone therapy for transmasculine persons consists of testosterone to develop secondary male sex characteristics.[3] In the skin, testosterone increases sebum production, increases facial and body hair growth, decreases scalp hair, and redistributes body fat (**Fig. 1**).[3] Gender-affirming hormone therapy for transfeminine persons consists of estrogen and/or antiandrogens, such as spironolactone, in the United States and cyproterone in most of Europe and gonadotropin-releasing hormone agonists in the United Kingdom.[4] In the skin, estrogen decreases skin sebum production, reduces facial and body hair growth, promotes epidermal thickness, stimulates melanocytes, and changes sweat and odor pattern.[3,5] Masculinizing and feminizing effects in the skin may be observed within 1 month of hormone therapy initiation but may not reach maximum effect until a few years later.[3]

COMMON SKIN CONDITIONS IN TRANSMASCULINE PERSONS
Acne Vulgaris

Acne vulgaris is a common and chronic skin disease characterized by the formation of comedones (blackheads and whiteheads), papules, pustules, nodules, and cysts.[6] Clogged hair follicles, increased skin sebum production, and the inflammatory response incited by Propionibacterium acnes contribute to the development of acne.[7] Acne is frequently driven by androgens.[8-10] Other risk factors may include chest binding, diet, stress, and medications—such as corticosteroids and lithium.[8,11]

Acne often has an impact on the psychosocial health of affected individuals.[12] Conspicuous acne lesions, secondary postinflammatory hyperpigmentation, and scars can be disfiguring and stigmatizing (**Fig. 2**). Patients with acne experience higher rates of low self-esteem, depression, and withdrawal from social activities and relationships.[13] A survey of 3775 18-year-old to 19 year-old young adults found those with significant acne were more likely to have suicidal ideation and mental health problems compared with those without acne.[14] Sexual minority patients with acne also were

Androgens

- Increase in sebaceous gland sebum production
- Increase in facial and body hair growth
- Decrease in scalp hair
- redistributed body fats

Estrogen

- Decrease in sebaceous gland sebum production
- Decrease in facial and body hair growth
- Increase in epidermal thickness
- Increase in melanocyte stimulation
- changed sweat and odor patterns

Fig. 1. Dermatologic effects of hormones.

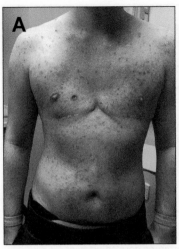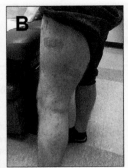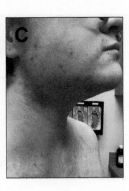

Fig. 2. Acne excoriée and pseudofolliculitis barbae in a transmasculine patient receiving testosterone. (*A*) Multiple erythematous papules and pustules, scars, and excoriated ulcer on the right chest. Linear scars denote prior chest surgery. (*B*) Erythematous crusted papules and pustules on the left leg. (*C*) Erythematous crusted papules and pustules on jawline worsened by hair plucking..

shown to have increased risks of suicidal ideation and antidepressant use compared with sexual minority patients without acne.[15]

High rates of acne with gender-affirming testosterone therapy has been noted.[11] For example, 1 study of 21 transmasculine adults found 94% had facial acne and 88% back acne after 4 months of testosterone therapy, an increase from pretreatment rates of 29% and 17%, respectively.[16] Although the natural history of hormone therapy–induced acne remains poorly understood, small studies suggest that acne severity often peaks in the first 6 months of testosterone therapy and may gradually improve over 1 year to 2 years.[17–19] The psychosocial effects of acne may compound gender dysphoria and high preexisting rates of psychiatric comorbidity in transgender patients.[20,21] Because clinicians often underestimate patients' negative experience and impact from acne, signs and symptoms of acne should be inquired about, addressed and treated if symptomatic, even if considered mild based on a clinician's initial impression.[21]

Acne severity should direct initial therapy (**Table 1**).[22] The Investigator Global Assessment severity scale (**Table 2**) is a commonly used tool to classify acne as clear, almost clear, mild, moderate, or severe. Acne with cysts, nodules, or significant scarring is often treated as severe.[22] First-line therapy for mild acne is a topical retinoid, topical benzoyl peroxide (BP), or a combination of the 2.[7] Topical retinoids, such as tretinoin, adapalene, and tazarotene, are comedolytic and anti-inflammatory agents that serve as the core of acne therapy.[7] They help resolve precursor microcomedone lesions and improve secondary scarring and hyperpigmentation.[23] Topical adapalene, 0.1% gel, is now available over the counter and may be considered for patients whose insurance plans do not cover topical retinoids. Common side effects of topical retinoids include photosensitivity, skin dryness, peeling, erythema, and irritation. Side effects are minimized by slow up-titration and typically peak in the first 2 weeks to 4 weeks of use, improving over time. Anticipatory guidance is crucial to improving adherence and preventing premature

Table 1
Initial treatment options for mild, moderate, and severe acne as adapted from the American Academy of Dermatology acne guidelines

Mild	Moderate	Severe
• Topical retinoid alone OR • Topical retinoid + BP OR • BP alone OR • BP + topical clindamycin/ erythromycin	• Combination topical retinoid + BP + topical clindamycin/ erythromycin OR • Oral antibiotics (eg, doxycycline, 100 mg bid, for no more than 3 mo, taper once improved) concurrent with topical retinoid ± BP	• Referral to dermatology for consideration of isotretinoin or other treatment options AND • Oral antibiotics (eg, doxycycline, 100 mg bid, for no more than 3 mo, taper once improved) concurrent with topical retinoid ± BP

Treat patient until clear or almost clear before tapering therapy. In cases of poor response to initial treatment, discuss acne triggers, medication side effects (eg, dryness and irritation), and adherence; consider referral to dermatology; and consider testosterone dose adjustment.[7]

treatment discontinuation.[23] Patients should be counseled to apply a small pea-size amount every 2 nights to 3 nights, then gradually increase frequency to nightly over 2 weeks to 4 weeks, as tolerated, with concurrent daily moisturizer and sunscreen use.[7] BP, available over the counter in 2.5% to 10% washes, creams, or gels, is effective for mild to moderate inflammatory acne. It can be used as monotherapy or in combination with various concentrations of topical clindamycin or erythromycin and/or topical retinoids. Current guidelines do not recommend topical antibiotic monotherapy without BP due to emerging bacterial resistance. For moderate acne, combination topical therapies with a combination of topical retinoids and/or topcial BP with or without topical antibiotics initially should be used. Systemic antibiotics, most commonly oral doxycycline or minocycline, also should be considered for moderate to severe acne. Oral antibiotics should be limited to the shortest possible duration (<3 months). Concurrent topical therapy is crucial to sustain acne improvement after antibiotic tapering. Patients with moderate to severe acne, as well as those with significant postinflammatory hyperpigmentation or scarring, should be referred to dermatology for aggressive treatment to prevent further scarring or disfiguration.

Table 2
Investigator global assessment scale for acne

Grade	Clinical Description
0 (clear)	No comedones (blackheads/whiteheads) or inflammatory papules/pustules
1 (almost clear)	Rare comedones with 1 to a few inflammatory papules/pustules
2 (mild)	Some comedones with no more than a few inflammatory papules/pustules; no nodules
3 (moderate)	Many comedones with some inflammatory papules/pustules; up to 1 small nodule
4 (severe)	Many comedones and inflammatory papules/pustules; more than 1 nodule

Data from Acne Vulgaris: Establishing Effectiveness of Drugs Intended for Treatment- Guidance for Industry. Food and Drug Administration, Center for Drug Evaluation and Research: 2018. Available at: fda.gov/downloads/drugs/guidances.

Oral isotretinoin has been effective at treating severe, refractory, or nodulocystic hormone-induced acne in transgender patients without interfering with testosterone dosing.[18] Isotretinoin is a potent teratogen and all US patients are required to registered in the iPLEDGE system by the US Food and Drug Administration (FDA). Isotretinoin patients with reproductive potential must concurrently use 2 forms of effective contraception and undergo monthly pregnancy tests and counseling with their isotretinoin prescriber. Unfortunately, iPLEDGE currently enforces a gender-binary patient classification system, requiring patients to be registered and provided contraception management based on gender assigned at birth rather than focusing on anatomic inventory and sexual behaviors with reproductive potential.[24] Gender-neutral reform of the iPLEDGE system has been advocated. Isotretinoin may be associated with increased risks of depression and suicidality as well as delayed surgical wound healing for up to 6 months to 12 months after isotretinoin completion. Multidisciplinary care coordination among dermatologists, mental health providers, gynecologists, endocrinologists, and/or surgeons is crucial.

MALE PATTERN HAIR LOSS/ANDROGENETIC ALOPECIA

Male pattern hair loss (MPHL), also known as androgenetic or androgenic alopecia, is the most common cause of progressive hair loss. The multifactorial causes include age, androgens, and genetic predisposition.[25] In cisgender men, MPHL is associated with anxiety, depression, and sexual dysfunction.[26]

MPHL is characterized by hair loss in the temporal scalp, midfrontal scalp, or vertex area of the scalp in a horseshoe pattern. The midoccipital region is mostly unaffected.[27] Circulating 5α-dihydrotestosterone (DHT), converted from testosterone by 5α-reductase, interacts with androgen receptors in hair follicles. DHT miniaturizes scalp hair follicles and shortens the anagen stage, that is, the primary growth stage of hair, resulting in progressively decreasing hair coverage of the scalp.[28] Concomitant nail pitting, scalp itch, or focal hair loss beyond the scalp vertex may warrant dermatology referral.[28]

Hormone-induced MPHL presents similarly in transmasculine patients as in cisgender men. It often begins a few years after initiation of testosterone.[17,29] A cross-sectional study of 50 transmasculine patients showed mild to severe hair-loss in 62% of the participants on long-term testosterone; only 1 transmasculine person acquired MPHL within the first year of therapy.[17] MPHL may be a desirable masculine feature for some TM patients, but unwanted by others.[30]

Topical minoxidil and oral finasteride are first-line therapies for MPHL.[29] Topical minoxidil (Rogaine, Johnson & Johnson), a potent vasodilator, is available over the counter for men as a 5% solution or foam. It is safe for long-term use and improves hair survival, increases the duration of the anagen growth phase, revitalizes hair-keratin proteins, and decreases inflammatory signals on the scalp.[31–33] In 1 study, 51% of patients noted benefit from 5% minoxidil compared with 26% with placebo and significantly higher hair count was noted in the minoxidil group.[34] Side effects may include scalp irritation, dryness, itching, and redness. Patients with MPHL refractory to minoxidil should be referred to a dermatologist for more extensive treatment. Oral finasteride, an FDA-approved treatment of MPHL, is a competitive inhibitor of type II 5α-reductase enzyme on hair follicles to inhibit conversion of testosterone to DHT. It improves scalp coverage in cisgender men; 1 meta-analysis suggested a 25% increase in hair counts.[26,35,36] It does not interfere with serum testosterone level in transmasculine patients but effects on secondary gender characteristics are still unclear.[30,37] Some investigators have suggested that finasteride should be delayed until all desired gender-affirming changes secondary to hormone therapy are complete (usually after 2 years of testosterone therapy).[30] Finasteride was safe and effective in 1 study of 10 transmasculine patients.[37] Side effects of finasteride may include teratogenicity, sexual dysfunction, depression, breast enlargement, and the potential to mask elevations in prostate-specific antigen.[25]

COMMON SKIN CONDITIONS IN TRANSFEMININE PERSONS
Hirsutism/Pseudofolliculitis Barbae

Estrogen and antiandrogen treatments generally do not cause cessation of facial hair growth.[38] Facial hair is visually prominent and common male secondary gender characteristic that is associated with body image dissatisfaction in transfeminine persons.[39] Facial hirsutism in transfeminine persons can be disfiguring and contribute to gender dysphoria. Hair removal is considered medically necessary for transfeminine persons suffering from associated gender dysphoria.[40] Additionally, hair removal is important prior to genital gender-affirming surgeries. Hair follicles on surgically inverted skin flaps can lead to postoperative intravaginal or intraurethral hair growth and serve as a nidus for irritation and infection.[30] Mild hirsutism can be treated with shaving, plucking, threading, waxing, or topical eflornithine (Vaniqa, Allergan), which is FDA approved to treat hirsutism in women. More permanent treatment options for facial hair and for preoperative skin flap hair removal include electrolysis and laser hair removal.

The frequent shaving or trimming of facial hair in transfeminine patients with hirsutism can lead to pseudofolliculitis barbae (PFB), also known as razor bumps. PFB is a common condition of the bearded area, axilla, pubic region, and legs.[41] It is a chronic inflammatory disorder that primarily affects individuals with curled hair. Prevalence rates reach 80% in African American and Hispanic cisgender men and cisgender women with facial hirsutism or hypertrichosis.[42,43] Curved hair can grow back into the skin after being shaved or trimmed, causing inflammation and a foreign body reaction.[43] This presents as painful, itchy papules with erythema and hyperpigmentation. Postinflammatory hyperpigmentation or keloid scarring may develop. Patients often find the disorder distressing, and it may exacerbate gender dysphoria.[43] Discontinuation of shaving typically is curative for PFB, but this is generally inappropriate for transfeminine persons. It can be alleviated with proper shaving techniques or use of topical depilatories. Preshave preparation with mild soap and warm water is recommended before applying shaving cream, followed by shaving in nonoverlapping and unidirectional strokes.[43] More likely, medical therapy is needed (**Box 1**). Topical retinoids and low-potency topical corticosteroid may be used as first-line therapy.[42]

Box 1
Summary of treatment options for pseudofolliculitis barbae

Default to more aggressive therapies due to the secondary scarring of PFB and the psychosocial toll of the condition in the transgender population:
- Depilatories
- Topical retinoids and low-potency topical corticosteroids
- Eflornithine (reduces hair growth)
- BP and/or topical clindamycin (decreases inflammatory lesions)
- Laser hair removal (destruction of hair follicle through laser of a wavelength primarily absorbed by melanin, which is concentrated in the hair follicle)
- Electrolysis (individual destruction of hair follicles with electrified probe)

Combination BP and topical clindamycin may also reduce inflammation and lesion count.[44] Eflornithine may be added to reduce hair growth.[42] Destruction of hair follicles through laser hair removal has become the gold standard for a permanent treatment option, although electrolysis can also be used.[45] PFB can be difficult to treat and early referral to dermatology should be considered to prevent postinflammatory hyperpigmentation and scarring.[4,29]

Complications from Dermal Fillers for Facial/Body Contouring

Facial feminization and body contouring procedures are common for transfeminine persons. Neuromodulators, such as botulinum toxin A injections and dermal fillers yield immediate and long-lasting contouring and feminizing effect. Transgender individuals often face barriers to care and are affected by the high cost of these procedures and are at risk to engage in unsafe practices, such as receiving fillers from unlicensed personnel.[46,47] Injections of illicit filler material by nonlicensed persons are often toxic with complications, including foreign-body granulomas; bacterial, fungal or mycobacterial infections; bleeding; pain; scarring and keloid formation; ulceration and necrosis; gross disfiguration; silicone embolism; and death **(Fig. 3)**.[46,47] Prevalence estimates of unlicensed silicone injections in the transfeminine population have ranged from 25% to 32%; this is of particular concern given the high complication rate of silicone injections.[48,49] Commonly used FDA-approved materials include collagen, hyaluronic acid, calcium hydroxylapatite, poly-L-lactic acid, and polymethylmethacrylate.[50] Physicians should refer patients to licensed physicians, such as board-certified dermatologists and plastic surgeons, for dermal fillers and to treat dermal complications from illicit filler use.[50]

Keloids and Hypertrophic Scars

Keloids and hypertrophic scars are fibrous proliferation initially caused by dermal injury.[51] Hypertrophic scars and keloids present as firm and elevated flesh-colored papules and nodules.[52] Hypertrophic scars remain within the borders of the original scar, whereas keloids extend beyond the original scar. They are occasionally pruritic or painful. The appearance and physical discomfort can have a significant impact on a patient's quality of life and can lead to depression and social withdrawal.[53]

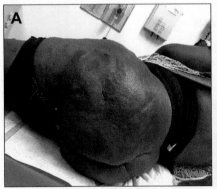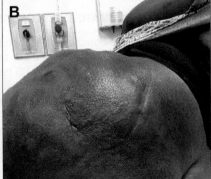

Fig. 3. (A) A transfeminine patient with painful plaques on bilateral buttocks years after illicit filler injections, complicated by pulmonary embolism. (B) Examination reveals hyperpigmented plaques that are firmly indurated and tender upon palpation.

Like all individuals undergoing surgery, transgender patients undergoing gender-affirming surgery are at risk for hypertrophic scar and keloid development, especially if they have a darker-skin type, have a family or personal history of keloids, or undergo surgery at high-tension skin areas, such as the chest.[54] Keloid scarring can hinder a transgender patients' ability to pass as their identified gender.[30] Keloids and hypertrophic scars usually develop over a period of weeks or months. Surgical scar prevention and management should be discussed in at-risk patients. These patients should be carefully monitored even several months after surgery.

The first-line therapy for both treatment and prevention of keloid and hypertrophic scars is intralesional corticosteroid injections.[52] Repeated triamcinolone injections yield moderate reduction of the scar with 50% reoccurrence rate a few years after injection.[55] Surgical excision is an option for treatment-resistant keloids, but there is a high risk of reoccurrence without both postoperative and follow-up injections of intralesional corticosteroids.[52] Dermatology referral is warranted given the often refractory or recurrent nature of keloids.

Melasma

Melasma, also known as chloasma, is a skin pigmentary disorder that affects 8% to 40% of the population and is one of the most frequent dermatologic complaints worldwide.[56] Melasma affects more than 5 million Americans of all skin types and ethnic groups. Higher prevalence is observed in population in intertropical areas where there is greater exposure to ultraviolet radiation, such as Washington, DC, and Texas, and those of skin types III, IV, and V.[57] Melasma can be disfiguring and impactful to a patient's social life and emotional well-being.[58]

Melasma presents as symmetric hyperpigmented brown to blueish-gray macules and patches on the sun-exposed skin, especially the face. Darker skin types, ultraviolet radiation exposure, and hormones, in particular estrogen, are risk factors for melasma.[59] There is no pain or other associated symptoms. Transfeminine patients undergoing estrogen hormone therapy are at risk of developing melasma. Melasma management includes prevention of further hyperpigmentation and lightening of affected skin. Strict use of sunscreen and photoprotection is required. Hydroquinone, 2% to 4% cream, is the first-line skin lightening agent and can be combined with topical retinoids or corticosteroids.[59] Dermatology referral is warranted for treatment of refractory melasma with additional treatment options such as chemical peels and lasers.

MISCELLANEOUS DERMATOLOGIC CONDITIONS

Another dermatologic condition described in transgender persons is lichen sclerosus. Lichen sclerosus presents as crinkled or thickened patches of skin with pruritus and tenderness at the anogenital area.[60] LS has been reported in transfeminine patients and ought to be treated and monitored.[61,62] Complications of lichen sclerosus may include scarring, pruritus, pain, and obliteration of external genitalia as well as squamous cell carcinoma.

Human papillomavirus (HPV) infection and HPV-related skin diseases also have occurred in the neovagina of transfeminine patients. These diseases include condylomas, which can be treated with topical application of trichloroacetic acid, cryotherapy, or surgical excision. Low-risk dysplasia, high-risk dysplasia, and HPV-related squamous cell carcinoma also all have been reported.[63,64]

The transgender population has increased prevalence of HIV rates and is subsequently at risk for HIV-associated dermatologic conditions.[65] HIV patients with normal

CD4 T-cell levels can develop psoriasis, folliculitis, condylomas, seborrheic dermatitis, and dry skin. Lower T-cell levels can predispose patients to basal cell carcinoma, squamous cell carcinoma, Kaposi sarcoma, resistant herpes simplex, molluscum contagiosum, fungal infection, and so forth.[65]

SUMMARY

Transgender persons face unique burdens of dermatologic conditions related to cutaneous effects of gender-affirming hormone therapy and procedures. Skin diseases in transgender patients often are underdiagnosed and underrecognized despite potential for significant impairments in quality of life and mental health from skin diseases. For transmasculine patients, common conditions include acne vulgaris and MPHL. For transfeminine patients, common conditions include hirsutism, PFB, and melasma. Postprocedural keloids and complications of filler injections should be considered. Unique aspects of skin health in transgender persons should be considered in the context of multidisciplinary gender-affirming care. Greater recognition and implementation of dermatologic care will improve overall clinical outcomes of gender-affirming care in transgender patients.

ACKNOWLEDGMENTS

Dr Yeung was supported in part by the Dermatology Foundation and the National Center for Advancing Translational Sciences (NCATS) of the National Institutes of Health under award number UL1TR002378 and KL2TR002381. The content is solely the responsibility of the authors and does not necessarily represent the official views of the National Institutes of Health.

REFERENCES

1. Owen-Smith AA, Gerth J, Sineath RC, et al. Association between gender confirmation treatments and perceived gender congruence, body image satisfaction, and mental health in a cohort of transgender individuals. J Sex Med 2018; 15(4):591–600.
2. Gonzales G, Henning-Smith C. Barriers to care among transgender and gender nonconforming adults. Milbank Q 2017;95(4):726–48.
3. Hembree WC, Cohen-Kettenis PT, Gooren L, et al. Endocrine treatment of gender-dysphoric/gender-incongruent persons: an endocrine society clinical practice guideline. J Clin Endocrinol Metab 2017;102(11):3869–903.
4. Center of Excellence for Transgender Health, Department of Family and Community Medicine, University of California San Francisco. In: Deutsch MB, editor. Guidelines for the Primary and Gender-Affirming Care of Transgender and Gender Nonbinary People. 2nd ed. San Francisco (CA): University of California, San Francisco; 2016.
5. Stevenson S, Thornton J. Effect of estrogens on skin aging and the potential role of SERMs. Clin Interv Aging 2007;2(3):283.
6. Zaenglein AL, Graber EM, Thiboutot DM. Acne vulgaris and acneiform eruptions. In: Goldsmith LA, Katz SI, Gilchrest BA, et al, editors. Fitzpatrick's dermatology in general medicine, 8e. New York: The McGraw-Hill Companies; 2012. p. 897–917.
7. Zaenglein AL, Pathy AL, Schlosser BJ, et al. Guidelines of care for the management of acne vulgaris. J Am Acad Dermatol 2016;74(5):945–73.e33.

8. Elsaie ML. Hormonal treatment of acne vulgaris: an update. Clin Cosmet Investig Dermatol 2016;9:241–8.

9. Trivedi MK, Shinkai K, Murase JE. A Review of hormone-based therapies to treat adult acne vulgaris in women. Int J Womens Dermatol 2017;3(1):44–52.

10. Ju Q, Tao T, Hu T, et al. Sex hormones and acne. Clin Dermatol 2017;35(2):130–7.

11. Motosko C, Zakhem G, Pomeranz M, et al. Acne: a side effect of masculinizing hormonal therapy in transgender patients. Br J Dermatol 2018;180(1):26–30.

12. Dalgard F, Gieler U, Holm JO, et al. Self-esteem and body satisfaction among late adolescents with acne: results from a population survey. J Am Acad Dermatol 2008;59(5):746–51.

13. Revol O, Milliez N, Gerard D. Psychological impact of acne on 21st-century adolescents: decoding for better care. Br J Dermatol 2015;172(Suppl 1):52–8.

14. Halvorsen JA, Stern RS, Dalgard F, et al. Suicidal ideation, mental health problems, and social impairment are increased in adolescents with acne: a population-based study. J Invest Dermatol 2011;131(2):363–70.

15. Gao Y, Wei EK, Arron ST, et al. Acne, sexual orientation, and mental health among young adults in the United States: a population-based, cross-sectional study. J Am Acad Dermatol 2017;77(5):971–3.

16. Giltay E, Gooren L. Effects of sex steroid deprivation/administration on hair growth and skin sebum production in transsexual males and females. J Clin Endocrinol Metab 2000;85(8):2913–21.

17. Wierckx K, Van de Peer F, Verhaeghe E, et al. Short- and long-term clinical skin effects of testosterone treatment in trans men. J Sex Med 2014;11(1):222–9.

18. Turrion-Merino L, Urech-García-de-la-Vega M, Miguel-Gomez L, et al. Severe acne in female-to-male transgender patients. JAMA Dermatol 2015;151(11):1260–1.

19. Permpongkosol S, Khupulsup K, Leelaphiwat S, et al. Effects of 8-year treatment of long-acting testosterone undecanoate on metabolic parameters, urinary symptoms, bone mineral density, and sexual function in men with late-onset hypogonadism. J Sex Med 2016;13(8):1199–211.

20. Veale JF, Watson RJ, Peter T, et al. Mental health disparities among canadian transgender youth. J Adolesc Health 2017;60(1):44–9.

21. Torjesen I. Managing acne female-to-male transgender persons 2018. Available at: http://www.dermatologytimes.com/article/managing-acne-female-male-transgender-persons. Accessed August 19, 2018.

22. Thiboutot DM, Dreno B, Abanmi A, et al. Practical management of acne for clinicians: an international consensus from the Global Alliance to Improve Outcomes in Acne. J Am Acad Dermatol 2018;78(2S1):S1–23.e21.

23. Leyden J, Stein-Gold L, Weiss J. Why topical retinoids are mainstay of therapy for acne. Dermatol Ther (Heidelb) 2017;7(3):293–304.

24. Yeung H, Chen SC, Katz KA, et al. Prescribing isotretinoin in the United States for transgender individuals: ethical considerations. J Am Acad Dermatol 2016;75(3):648–51.

25. Kelly Y, Blanco A, Tosti A. Androgenetic alopecia: an update of treatment options. Drugs 2016;76(14):1349–64.

26. Tas B, Kulacaoglu F, Belli H, et al. The tendency towards the development of psychosexual disorders in androgenetic alopecia according to the different stages of hair loss: a cross-sectional study. An Bras Dermatol 2018;93(2):185–90.

27. Otberg N, Shapiro J. Hair growth disorders. In: Goldsmith LA, Katz SI, Gilchrest BA, et al, editors. Fitzpatrick's dermatology in general medicine, 8e. New York: The McGraw-Hill Companies; 2012. p. 979–1008.

28. Bolognia JL, Schaffer JV, Duncan KO, et al. Alopecias. Dermatology essentials. 1st edition. Philadelphia: Saunders; 2014.
29. Gao Y, Maurer T, Mirmirani P. Understanding and addressing hair disorders in transgender individuals. Am J Clin Dermatol 2018;19(4):517–27.
30. Ginsberg BA. Dermatologic care of the transgender patient. Int J Womens Dermatol 2017;3(1):65–7.
31. Civatte JC, Laux B, Simpson NB, et al. 2% topical minoxidil solution in male-pattern baldness: preliminary European results. Dermatology 1987;175(Suppl. 2):42–9.
32. Kanti V, Hillmann K, Kottner J, et al. Effect of minoxidil topical foam on frontotemporal and vertex androgenetic alopecia in men: a 104-week open-label clinical trial. J Eur Acad Dermatol Venereol 2016;30(7):1183–9.
33. Mirmirani P, Consolo M, Oyetakin-White P, et al. Similar response patterns to topical minoxidil foam 5% in frontal and vertex scalp of men with androgenetic alopecia: a microarray analysis. Br J Dermatol 2015;172(6):1555–61.
34. Olsen EA, Dunlap FE, Funicella T, et al. A randomized clinical trial of 5% topical minoxidil versus 2% topical minoxidil and placebo in the treatment of androgenetic alopecia in men. J Am Acad Dermatol 2002;47(3):377–85.
35. Choudhry R, Hodgins MB, Van der Kwast TH, et al. Localization of androgen receptors in human skin by immunohistochemistry: implications for the hormonal regulation of hair growth, sebaceous glands and sweat glands. J Endocrinol 1992;133(3):467–75.
36. Mella JM, Perret MC, Manzotti M, et al. Efficacy and safety of finasteride therapy for androgenetic alopecia: a systematic review. Arch Dermatol 2010;146(10):1141–50.
37. Moreno-Arrones OM, Becerra A, Vano-Galvan S. Therapeutic experience with oral finasteride for androgenetic alopecia in female-to-male transgender patients. Clin Exp Dermatol 2017;42(7):743–8.
38. Hembree WC, Cohen-Kettenis P, Delemarre-van de Waal HA, et al. Endocrine treatment of transsexual persons: an Endocrine Society clinical practice guideline. J Clin Endocrinol Metab 2009;94(9):3132–54.
39. van de Grift TC, Cohen-Kettenis PT, Steensma TD, et al. Body satisfaction and physical appearance in gender dysphoria. Arch Sex Behav 2016;45(3):575–85.
40. World Professional Association for Transgender Health. WPATH recommended benefits policy document: created in partnership with starbucks. Available at: https://www.wpath.org/media/cms/Documents/Public%20Policies/2018/6_June/Transgender%20Medical%20Benefits.pdf. Accessed August 19, 2018.
41. Bridgeman-Shah S. The medical and surgical therapy of pseudofolliculitis barbae. Dermatol Ther 2004;17(2):158–63.
42. Perry PK, Cook-Bolden FE, Rahman Z, et al. Defining pseudofolliculitis barbae in 2001: a review of the literature and current trends. J Am Acad Dermatol 2002;46(2):S113–9.
43. Agi C, Bosley RE. Pseudofolliculitis barbae and acne keloidalis nuchae. In: Aguh C, Okoye GA, editors. Fundamentals of ethnic hair: the dermatologist's perspective. Cham (Switzerland): Springer International Publishing; 2017. p. 123–33.
44. Cook-Bolden FE, Barba A, Halder R, et al. Twice-daily applications of benzoyl peroxide 5%/clindamycin 1% gel versus vehicle in the treatment of pseudofolliculitis barbae. Cutis 2004;73(6 Suppl):18–24.
45. Xia Y, Cho S, Howard RS, et al. Topical eflornithine hydrochloride improves the effectiveness of standard laser hair removal for treating pseudofolliculitis barbae: a randomized, double-blinded, placebo-controlled trial. J Am Acad Dermatol 2012;67(4):694–9.

46. Wilson E, Rapues J, Jin H, et al. The use and correlates of illicit silicone or "fillers" in a population-based sample of transwomen, San Francisco, 2013. J Sex Med 2014;11(7):1717–24.

47. Clark K, Fletcher JB, Holloway IW, et al. Structural inequities and social networks impact hormone use and misuse among transgender women in Los Angeles county. Arch Sex Behav 2018;47(4):953–62.

48. Herbst JH, Jacobs ED, Finlayson TJ, et al. Estimating HIV prevalence and risk behaviors of transgender persons in the United States: a systematic review. AIDS Behav 2008;12(1):1–17.

49. Sevelius JM. Gender affirmation: a framework for conceptualizing risk behavior among transgender women of color. Sex Roles 2013;68(11–12):675–89.

50. U.S. Food & Drug Administration. Dermal fillers (soft tissue fillers) - dermal fillers approved by the center for devices and radiological health. Available at: https://www.fda.gov/MedicalDevices/ProductsandMedicalProcedures/CosmeticDevices/ucm619846.htm. Accessed August 19, 2018.

51. Ogawa R. Keloid and hypertrophic scars are the result of chronic inflammation in the reticular dermis. Int J Mol Sci 2017;18(3) [pii:E606].

52. Chike-Obi CJ, Cole PD, Brissett AE. Keloids: pathogenesis, clinical features, and management. Semin Plast Surg 2009;23(3):178–84.

53. Walliczek U, Engel S, Weiss C, et al. Clinical outcome and quality of life after a multimodal therapy approach to ear keloids. JAMA Facial Plast Surg 2015; 17(5):333–9.

54. Hage JJ, van Kesteren PJ. Chest-wall contouring in female-to-male transsexuals: basic considerations and review of the literature. Plast Reconstr Surg 1995;96(2): 386–91.

55. Trisliana Perdanasari A, Torresetti M, Grassetti L, et al. Intralesional injection treatment of hypertrophic scars and keloids: a systematic review regarding outcomes. Burns Trauma 2015;3:14.

56. Handel AC, Miot LDB, Miot HA. Melasma: a clinical and epidemiological review. An Bras Dermatol 2014;89(5):771–82.

57. Davis EC, Callender VD. Postinflammatory hyperpigmentation. J Clin Aesthet Dermatol 2010;3(7):20–31.

58. Balkrishnan R, McMichael AJ, Camacho FT, et al. Development and validation of a health-related quality of life instrument for women with melasma. Br J Dermatol 2003;149(3):572–7.

59. Halder RM, Nootheti PK. Ethnic skin disorders overview. J Am Acad Dermatol 2003;48(6 Suppl):S143–8.

60. Tasker GL, Wojnarowska F. Lichen sclerosus. Clin Exp Dermatol 2003;28(2):128–33.

61. McMurray SL, Overholser E, Patel T. A transgender woman with anogenital lichen sclerosus. JAMA Dermatol 2017;153(12):1334–5.

62. Amend B, Seibold J, Toomey P, et al. Surgical reconstruction for male-to-female sex reassignment. Eur Urol 2013;64(1):141–9.

63. van der Sluis WB, Buncamper ME, Bouman MB, et al. Symptomatic HPV-related neovaginal lesions in transgender women: case series and review of literature. Sex Transm Infect 2016;92(7):499–501.

64. Bollo J, Balla A, Rodriguez Luppi C, et al. HPV-related squamous cell carcinoma in a neovagina after male-to-female gender confirmation surgery. Int J STD AIDS 2018;29(3):306–8.

65. Radix A, Sevelius J, Deutsch MB. Transgender women, hormonal therapy and HIV treatment: a comprehensive review of the literature and recommendations for best practices. J Int AIDS Soc 2016;19(3 Suppl 2):20810.

Cancer Risk in Transgender People

Christel J.M. de Blok, MD[a,b], Koen M.A. Dreijerink, MD, PhD[a,b],
Martin den Heijer, MD, PhD[a,b],*

KEYWORDS

- Transgender • Cancer • Sex hormones • Sex differences

KEY POINTS

- Hormonal treatment in transgender people may affect sex-hormone related cancer risk, but reliable epidemiologic data are sparse.
- Based on the available data, the observed cancer risk in transgender people does not exceed known differences in cancer risk between cis- men and -women.
- Transgender people may develop cancer in organs that are related to their sex assigned at birth as well as in newly formed organs.
- The authors recommend cancer screening according to local guidelines for the organs present.

INTRODUCTION

The risk of certain types of cancer differs between men and women. This is obvious for cancers that develop in sex-specific organs such as the breast, cervix, and prostate, but cancer incidences of other types of cancer differ between sexes as well. Some of these differences are attributed to exposure to sex hormones, especially estrogen and testosterone. Transgender people, defined as an incongruence between one's sex assigned at birth and one's experienced gender identity, often seek (medical) care including gender-affirming hormone treatment (HT). Although HT is considered safe in general, the question regarding (long-term) risk on sex hormone-related cancer remains. With increasing numbers of transgender people receiving HT, and increasing follow-up of these people, more data become available to assess cancer risk in transgender people. In this overview, cancer risk in transgender people and the implications for treatment and screening are reviewed. The following topics are discussed:

Disclosure Summary: The authors report no conflict of interest.
[a] Department of Internal Medicine, Amsterdam UMC, VU University Medical Center, Amsterdam, the Netherlands; [b] Center of Expertise on Gender Dysphoria, Amsterdam UMC, VU University Medical Center, PO Box 7057, 1007 MB Amsterdam, the Netherlands
* Corresponding author. Department of Internal Medicine, Section Endocrinology, Amsterdam UMC, VU University Medical Center, PO Box 7057, 1007 MB Amsterdam, the Netherlands.
E-mail address: m.denheijer@vumc.nl

Endocrinol Metab Clin N Am 48 (2019) 441–452
https://doi.org/10.1016/j.ecl.2019.02.005   **endo.theclinics.com**

sex differences in cancer, the complexity of cancer risk in transgender people, sex hormones as carcinogens, incidence studies (breast cancer, cancer of the male reproductive organs, cancer of the female reproductive organs, benign brain tumors, cancer related to sexually transmitted infections, other types of cancer), cancer treatment in transgender people, implications for cancer screening and prevention, and the article ends with a summary.

SEX DIFFERENCES IN CANCER

It is well known that cancer risks of different types of cancer differ between men and women. These differences are thought to be multifactorial, but are in the first place determined by the presence of the specific organ. Because much of the knowledge used in transgender health care is derived from studies performed in cisgender populations, it is important to understand the current knowledge of sex differences on cancer risk and survival in general before one can understand cancer risk in transgender people. An accessible source of cancer incidence statistics are national cancer registries, which report trends on cancer incidences and outcomes. The Global Initiative for Cancer Registry Development is an international partnership that provides cancer incidence and mortality estimations of 36 cancer types in 185 countries, the GLOBOCAN estimations. Their latest data showed that prostate cancer was the second most incident cancer in men and that breast cancer was the most commonly diagnosed cancer in women.[1] Compared with women, men were more susceptible to lung, liver, and skin cancer, and women were more susceptible to thyroid, breast, and adrenal cortex cancer compared with men.[2] Obviously, prostate and testicular cancers are specific for men and cervical, uterine, and ovarian cancers are specific for women.

However, not only incidence rates may differ between men and women, also survival rates may be different. Overall, men seem to have a lower cancer survival rate than women, especially for cancers of the breast, stomach and esophagus, lung, colorectum, and melanoma.[2-4] On the other hand, cancer survival rates were lower for bladder and renal cancer, and sarcoma in women compared with men.[2,3] Furthermore, differences between sexes regarding clinical presentation and treatment outcomes for several types of cancer have been reported.[5,6] The question why there is a difference in cancer incidence, survival, clinical presentation, and treatment outcomes for different types of cancer between men and women, remains largely unanswered. The most likely explanation is the difference in concentrations of circulating sex hormones. However, differences in lifestyle (eg, smoking habits and alcohol consumption), age at diagnosis, (cancer driver) genes, and sex-chromosomes also may play a role.[7-9] Moreover, it is important to realize that available incidence and survival data are largely based on data from high-income countries, because low- and middle-income countries often do not have high-quality cancer registries.[1]

THE COMPLEXITY OF CANCER RISK IN TRANSGENDER PEOPLE

The complex interaction between sex and cancer incidence and outcome becomes even more complex in transgender people. In transgender people receiving HT, circulating sex hormones are changed from sex hormones that belong to their sex assigned at birth to sex hormones belonging to their experienced gender. In transwomen (male sex assigned at birth, female gender identity), HT consists of estrogen treatment often combined with anti-androgens, some of which also have progestogenic properties. Transmen (female sex assigned at birth, male gender identity) are treated with testosterone. These (exogenous) hormones may not only affect the risk for sex-specific cancers, but also for other types of cancer that may contain receptors for sex hormones.

Fig. 1 shows an overview of different factors that may have an effect on cancer risk in transgender people. As depicted, besides sex hormones, the presence of certain organs is also an important factor in cancer risk of sex-specific cancers. Transwomen, for example, often undergo vaginoplasty as part of their transition, during which the testes are removed. The prostate, however, remains preserved, because removal of the prostate is associated with a high chance of urologic complications such as incontinence. Most transmen undergo a mastectomy (in literature also referred to as chest surgery), but the wish for an oophorectomy and/or hysterectomy varies across countries and over time. The change in surgery wishes over time and difference between countries may be partly explained by differences and changes in laws, for instance whether or not sterilization is required to change one's legal sex. Besides removal of organs, transgender people may undergo surgery that constructs new organs such as a neovagina in transwomen or a neophallus in transmen, leading to new possible cancer sites.

Not only hormones, surgery, and genes (which is discussed later) may have an effect on cancer risk in transgender people, also lifestyle factors, such as obesity, smoking habits, alcohol use, and sexual risk behavior, might play a role. Lifestyle may vary between transgender and cisgender people and between countries, depending on the marginalization of transgender people. The literature is inconsistent about whether these factors differ between transgender and cisgender people.[10–12]

Better defined cancer risk factors, are some sexually transmitted infections (STIs), such as human papillomavirus (HPV) and human immunodeficiency virus (HIV). The incidence of STIs may differ between countries and between cisgender and transgender people. Especially in transgender people who work as sex workers the incidence of STI may be increased.

The relation between sex and cancer risk is already multiform and complex. However, cancer risk in transgender people is even more complex, because all the above-described factors may not only act independently on cancer risk in transgender people, but may also show complex interactions. However, the available information and knowledge is poor. Registration of legal sex changes in national cancer registries is nearly absent or unreliable,[13] and the number of people in specific transgender registries are low and often lack long-term follow-up. Therefore, caution is needed when considering cancer risk in transgender people.[14]

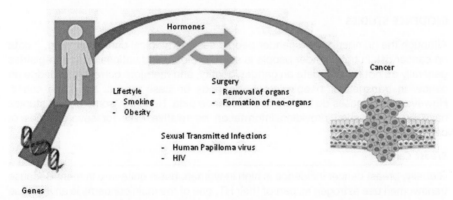

Fig. 1. Cancer risk in transgender people may be influenced by several factors, including genes, hormonal treatment, lifestyle factors, sexually transmitted infections, and surgical procedures.

SEX HORMONES AS CARCINOGENS

Through their receptors, sex hormones are involved in proliferative signaling and growth suppression in cells, 2 major underlying mechanisms of carcinogenesis.[15] Sex hormones may either play carcinogenic or tumor-suppressive roles. Whereas the role of estrogens, progestogens, and androgens has been comprehensively studied in breast cancer and prostate cancer in cisgender people, only in recent years are reports addressing this topic emerging in transgender research. The effects of gonadotropin-releasing hormone agonists and gonadectomy on cancer risk in transgender people have been explored to a very limited extent. DNA mutational landscapes in cancer have been reported to vary significantly between men and women.[9] However, there are no published studies addressing the role of such sex-dependent autosomal differences or sex chromosome-specific oncogenes or tumor suppressor genes and the risk of tumors that are typical for the assigned gender.

Estrogen receptor (ER) alpha is a major factor in the diagnosis and treatment of 70% of female breast cancer cases. Similar observations have been made in cisgender male breast cancer.[16] Most breast tumors in transwomen are of luminal type, expressing ER and/or the progesterone receptor (PR). Estrogens seems to be mainly important for breast cancer progression in cisgender women, supported by the results of The Women's Health Initiative trial, which demonstrated that combined use of estrogen and progestin in post-menopausal women resulted in a higher incidence of invasive breast cancer. However, use of estrogen alone did not increase this risk, suggesting a dominant role for progestogens in tumor initiation.[17] As cyproterone acetate, a PR-agonist, is used in Europe as anti-androgen in transwomen, this observation may be relevant for breast cancer development in transwomen. Further comparative studies are warranted to evaluate the use of PR-agonists and breast cancer risk in transwomen.

The androgen receptor (AR) is expressed in most female and male breast tumors, and seems to have dual roles in breast carcinogenesis in cisgender women. In luminal tumors, AR has growth suppressive properties, whereas in ER-negative breast cancers AR functions as a driver of tumor cell proliferation.[18] This may be of particular relevance for breast cancer arising in remnant breast tissue after subcutaneous mastectomy in transmen receiving HT. Moreover, activation of AR signaling is essential for prostate cancer growth. Depletion of testosterone levels and disruption of AR function is the mainstay of prostate cancer treatment in cisgender men.

INCIDENCE STUDIES

Although the number of transgender people seeking medical care is growing,[19] data on cancer risk in transgender people is scarce. Global and national cancer registries generally do not register data on gender identity, and therefore current knowledge on cancer in transgender people largely depends on case reports and case series. However, these cases do not provide incidence data. Recently, some cohort studies have been published providing information on relative risks for several types of cancers.[20–29]

Breast Cancer

Globally, breast cancer incidence is high in women, but is quite rare in men. Because transwomen use estrogen as part of their HT, one of the main concerns is an increase in breast cancer risk. Earlier reports showed a low number of breast cancer cases, leading to the opinion that breast cancer risk of transwomen receiving HT was comparable with the risk in cisgender men.[28] A recent study, however, showed a

46-fold increased risk of breast cancer in transwomen compared with reference men.[30] Furthermore, an interesting observation is that breast cancer in transwomen occurs at a younger age compared with cisgender women and occurs after a relatively short HT duration. Despite the fact that these new observations challenge established knowledge, the follow-up of all studies performed remain relatively short. Moreover, little is known about the cause of the increase in breast cancer risk in transwomen. A possible explanation may be genetic susceptibility; nevertheless further research should be performed to study these remaining questions. Moreover, in the literature, there is evidence that both testosterone and estrogen may play a role in breast cancer risk. Testosterone is thought to have a protective effect, and estrogen a stimulating effect. Because transwomen are commonly treated with both estrogen and anti-androgens, the increase of circulating estrogen and loss of circulating testosterone could contribute to the observed increased breast cancer risk compared with cisgender men.[18]

Cancer of the Male Reproductive Organs

An important question is whether HT induces an increase in cancer risk for the male reproductive organs. Under the influence of testosterone, the prostate is embryologically formed from the mesonephric duct (also known as the Wolffian duct), and is specific for men. As described above, the prostate is preserved in transwomen, even after vaginoplasty. Therefore, these individuals might still be at risk for prostate cancer. Only one study provides incidence data on prostate cancer in transgender people, and reported one case in 2306 transwomen followed for a total of 51,173 person years.[27] A recent literature review described 10 prostate cancer cases in transwomen worldwide.[31] This indicates that prostate cancer risk in transwomen is lower than in cisgender men, which may be explained by the anti-androgenic effect of HT and orchiectomy during vaginoplasty, both leading to low circulating testosterone levels. However, 6 of the 10 reported cases had metastases at time of diagnosis,[31] indicating either a delay in diagnosis or a more aggressive form of prostate cancer in transwomen. The role of estrogen in prostate cancer is unclear. On the one hand, prostate cancer cells might have ERs through which estrogen might induce prostate cancer in the presence of testosterone.[32] On the other hand, estrogens also may contribute to the low prostate cancer incidence in transwomen through the growth inhibitory actions of the ER beta or estrogen-related receptors.[33]

No incidence studies have been performed on testicular cancer in transwomen; in fact, only one case report has been described in the literature.[34]

Cancer of the Female Reproductive Organs

As in male reproductive cancer, the question is whether testosterone treatment increases the risk of cancer of the female reproductive organs in transmen. There is little evidence for a relation between testosterone treatment and ovarian cancer. Olsen and colleagues[35] showed an increased ovarian cancer risk in cisgender women with a history of testosterone treatment; however, the implications of this finding for transmen are unclear. All the more because follow-up of transmen receiving testosterone treatment and who still have their ovaries is small, since sterilization was required in many countries, and in some it still is, to be able to change one's legal sex. The largest study to date is performed by Grynberg and colleagues,[36] who studied the ovaries of 112 transmen who underwent hystero-salpingo-oophorectomy. They observed that mean ovarian volume was increased, with histopathological characteristics of polycystic ovaries in 89 transmen. They did not find any ovarian cancer case. Nevertheless, to date 6 case reports of transmen with ovarian cancer have been published.[37–40]

In the study of Grynberg and colleagues,[36] endometrial atrophy was observed in 45% of the investigated cases, but no cases of uterine cancer were seen. In the literature, only one case of uterine cancer in a transman has been described.[41] Minimal changes in cervical histology were observed in the study by Grynberg and colleagues;[36] cervical dysplasia was present in one case. Because cervical cancer is strongly related to HPV, this topic is further discussed in the context of STIs.

One case of vaginal cancer in a transman, who did not receive HT, has been described.[42] Two case-control studies compared vaginal biopsies from 16 transmen receiving HT with those of 32 cisgender women, in whom no cases of vaginal cancer were found.[43,44]

An increase in the number of transmen who will keep their (female) reproductive organs is expected over the following years. Therefore, long-term follow-up studies are needed to study cancer risk in these people.

Benign Brain Tumors; Pituitary Adenoma, Meningioma, and Vestibular Schwannoma

Meningioma, vestibular schwannoma, and pituitary adenomas, such as nonsecretive adenomas, prolactinomas, somatotrophinomas, corticotrophinomas, and thyrotrophinomas, are the most common benign brain tumors. Sex differences in the incidence of these brain tumors have been described in literature, and might be caused by differences in sex hormones or sex hormone receptors.[45–47] Therefore, an altered risk in transgender people receiving HT could be expected. Since estrogens stimulate prolactin production in the pituitary, one of the concerns of estrogen use in transwomen is an increased risk of prolactinomas. However, the literature is sparse. Several case reports on prolactinomas in transwomen have been published, but only one study provides incidence data.[48] This study showed an increased prolactinoma risk in transwomen compared with control men and women. Knowledge about other pituitary adenomas, meningiomas, and vestibular schwannomas is mostly retrieved from case reports. Nota and colleagues,[48] also reported the incidence of these tumors in their above-described study, and found an increased meningioma incidence in transwomen compared with a European female and male population. An interesting finding and possible explanation for this increased risk was that most transwomen still used cyproterone acetate at time of meningioma diagnosis, even after orchiectomy.[49] Furthermore, in transmen they observed an unexplained 22-fold increased risk of somatotrophinomas compared with a general European population.

Cancer Related to Sexually Transmitted Infections

Several STIs have been associated with an increased risk on specific types of cancer. The prevalence of STIs in transgender people may vary between different countries. Moreover, it differs in people depending on lifestyle factors, such as sexual risk behavior. For cervical cancer, there is a strong association with several types of HPV. As described above, minimal cervical histology changes have been described in transmen, and cervical dysplasia was rare in the study of Grynberg and colleagues.[36] Nevertheless, 3 case reports of transmen with cervical cancer have been described.[39,41,50] Unfortunately, in none of these cases was HPV status reported. Human papillomavirus is not only associated with cervical cancer, but also with anal and penile cancer. Despite the high prevalence of anal HPV among transwomen[51–54] in both sex workers[55] and non-sex workers,[56] vaccination rates remain low. A higher proportional incidence was found for anal cancer in transgender people compared with controls of the New York State Cancer Registry,[57] of whom most cases were HPV positive. The risk was not calculated for transwomen and transmen separately. No cases of penile cancer in transwomen have been reported.

Although chronic hepatitis B and C infections can cause hepatocellular carcinoma, no cases in transgender people have been described.

The prevalence of HIV among transgender people is studied extensively, but is not discussed here. People with HIV/AIDS have an increased risk of developing Kaposi sarcoma, non-Hodgkin's lymphoma (mostly primary central nervous system lymphoma, primary effusion lymphoma, or aggressive large B cell lymphomas), and cervical cancer. Hutchison and colleagues[57] found an increased proportional incidence rate for Kaposki sarcoma and non-Hodgkin's lymphoma among transgender people, as well as other non-HIV/AIDS-related types of cancer. However, analyses were not adjusted for comorbidity or HIV status.

Other Types of Cancer

Several studies investigated cancer prevalence in transgender people and found no overall increased cancer risk.[20–22,24,25] Asscheman and colleagues[20] did find an increased risk of lung and hematological cancer in transwomen, but the overall cancer risk was not increased. Despite there is no increased cancer risk found in transgender people, several cases have been described in literature, including lung cancer, hematological cancers, cancers of the gastrointestinal tract, brain tumors, melanomas, and liver and pancreatic cancers.[20–25] Unfortunately, the numbers are too small to derive firm conclusions. Some case reports have been published on cancer in newly (surgically) formed organs such as the neovagina in transwomen.[58,59] Although no incidence data are available here, the incidence seems very low. Nevertheless, it is important to keep in mind that cancer can occur in newly formed organs as well.

CANCER TREATMENT IN TRANSGENDER PEOPLE

Because there is no literature on cancer treatment outcomes in transgender people specifically, there is no knowledge on whether cancer treatment in transgender people should be different from treatment in cisgender people. Although a cancer diagnosis leads to significant fears and concerns, thereby affecting the well-being in all people affected, in transgender people cancer diagnosis in a sex-specific organ may cause extra distress. Furthermore, it should be kept in mind that people in the environment might not always know that someone is transgender. This should be discussed with the transgender person privately, before diagnosis and treatment options are discussed with family present.

When a hormone-sensitive/hormone-receptor-positive tumor is diagnosed, the question of whether or not to withdraw HT arises. This decision has to be balanced between the risk of progression or recurrence of the tumor on the one hand, and (further) increasing distress on the other hand, because HT in transgender people is very important for maintaining secondary sex characteristics and for psychological well-being. For comparison, the decision to withdraw HT in transwomen is as difficult for transwomen as the decision of whether to undergo an oophorectomy is for cisgender women.[60] Therefore, lowering the dose of HT could be a good compromise between cancer risk and maintaining effects on secondary sex characteristics, as the desired effects of HT also might be apparent at lower dosages. Moreover (cancer) health care providers need to show that they welcome (gender) diversity to be able to discuss openly treatment options, including lowering or withdrawing HT.

Considering the above-described, it might be clear that, in the care for transgender people with cancer, one must strive for a good balance between treatment and progression or recurrence risk on the one hand and the wishes and well-being of the affected person on the other, just as in any person with cancer.

IMPLICATIONS FOR CANCER SCREENING AND PREVENTION

In many countries, population cancer screening programs are available, including screening for breast and cervical cancer, and in some countries for prostate cancer as well. Usually, people are invited to participate based on registered sex and age in national or municipal registries. These registries, however, rarely register transition status and therefore fail to reach people who have changed their legal sex. This is not a problem when the specific organ has been removed, but is the more important in people who changed their legal sex and who still have the specific organ that is screened.

In transwomen, based on the current knowledge and the incidences described above, it seems reasonable to refer transwomen to participate in the population screening for breast cancer in the same schedule as cisgender women.[61,62] The need for screening for prostate cancer has been extensively studied in cisgender men. Although screening induces a slight reduction in prostate cancer-related mortality, it has also many disadvantages because of the relatively high false-positive rate.[63] Overall there is no strong support for prostate-specific antigen (PSA)-based prostate cancer screening.[64] When health care providers choose to determine PSA levels in transwomen receiving HT, they should know that the levels are probably much lower than in cisgender men because of low testosterone levels under anti-androgen treatment as part of HT. Since population-based prostate cancer screening is not generally implemented, and the incidence of prostate cancer seems much lower in transwomen than in cisgender men, there seems no reason to refer transwomen for regular prostate screening or perform regular PSA level measurements. However, health care providers and transwomen themselves should be aware that transwomen still have their prostate, even after vaginoplasty, and should consider prostate cancer, especially if a transwoman presents with lower urinary tract symptoms or hematuria.

In transmen, participation in the population-based screening for cervical cancer is indicated when the uterus is still present.[65] Recently, the feasibility of other approaches than the standard health care provider performed Pap-smear test, including self-testing, has been studied in transmen and might be a promising alternative.[66]

Although, an increased risk for meningiomas and prolactinomas in transwomen and somatotrophinomas in transmen has been described, these conditions are quite rare, so regular screenings for these tumors (eg, regular prolactin measurements for identifying prolactinomas) seem not to be indicated.

HPV vaccination is recommended for transwomen and transmen given the increased incidence of anal cancer,[67] and increasing awareness of the risks is necessary.[68]

Given all information available, there seems no need for intensified screening in transgender people for breast cancer, cervical cancer, prostate cancer, meningiomas, or prolactinomas. However, awareness, especially in transgender people, of the available population screening programs, is needed. Health care providers and policy-makers should ensure that transgender people have the opportunity to participate in population screening programs. Furthermore, health care providers should educate transgender people about current knowledge on screening and vaccination (e.g., HPV) programs, because many transgender people are not aware of the importance and availability of screening programs.[69]

SUMMARY

In summary, HT in transgender people may affect sex hormone-related cancer risk, but reliable epidemiologic data are sparse. The available data do not show an increased cancer risk in transgender people, and, more importantly, the observed risks do not exceed the risks seen in the general male and female populations. However, transgender people may develop cancer in organs that are related to their sex assigned at birth (prostate, cervix, breasts) as well as in newly formed organs (neovagina or neophallus). We recommend cancer screening according to local guidelines for the organs present. When cancer is diagnosed, a careful consideration of whether or not to withdraw HT should be made by both the treating health care providers and the affected transgender person.

REFERENCES

1. Bray F, Ferlay J, Soerjomataram I, et al. Global cancer statistics 2018: GLOBO-CAN estimates of incidence and mortality worldwide for 36 cancers in 185 countries. CA Cancer J Clin 2018;68(6):394–424.

2. Huang X, Shu C, Chen L, et al. Impact of sex, body mass index and initial pathologic diagnosis age on the incidence and prognosis of different types of cancer. Oncol Rep 2018;40(3):1359–69.

3. Afshar N, English DR, Thursfield V, et al. Differences in cancer survival by sex: a population-based study using cancer registry data. Cancer Causes Control 2018; 29(11):1059–69.

4. Wainer Z, Wright GM, Gough K, et al. Sex-dependent staging in non-small-cell lung cancer; analysis of the effect of sex differences in the eighth edition of the tumor, node, metastases staging system. Clin Lung Cancer 2018;19(6):e933–44.

5. Koo JH, Leong RW. Sex differences in epidemiological, clinical and pathological characteristics of colorectal cancer. J Gastroenterol Hepatol 2010;25(1):33–42.

6. Waldhoer T, Berger I, Haidinger G, et al. Sex differences of >/= pT1 bladder cancer survival in Austria: a descriptive, long-term, nation-wide analysis based on 27,773 patients. Urol Int 2015;94(4):383–9.

7. Arnold AP, Cassis LA, Eghbali M, et al. Sex hormones and sex chromosomes cause sex differences in the development of cardiovascular diseases. Arterioscler Thromb Vasc Biol 2017;37(5):746–56.

8. Spatz A, Borg C, Feunteun J. X-chromosome genetics and human cancer. Nat Rev Cancer 2004;4(8):617–29.

9. Li CH, Haider S, Shiah YJ, et al. Sex differences in cancer driver genes and biomarkers. Cancer Res 2018;78(19):5527–37.

10. Van Caenegem E, Taes Y, Wierckx K, et al. Low bone mass is prevalent in male-to-female transsexual persons before the start of cross-sex hormonal therapy and gonadectomy. Bone 2013;54(1):92–7.

11. Van Caenegem E, Wierckx K, Taes Y, et al. Body composition, bone turnover, and bone mass in trans men during testosterone treatment: 1-year follow-up data from a prospective case-controlled study (ENIGI). Eur J Endocrinol 2015;172(2): 163–71.

12. King BA, Dube SR, Tynan MA. Current tobacco use among adults in the United States: findings from the national adult tobacco survey. Am J Public Health 2012;102(11):e93–100.

13. Cathcart-Rake EJ, Lightner DJ, Quevedo FJ, et al. Cancer in transgender patients: one case in 385,820 is indicative of a paucity of data. J Oncol Pract 2018;14(4):270–2.

14. Braun H, Nash R, Tangpricha V, et al. Cancer in transgender people: evidence and methodological considerations. Epidemiol Rev 2017;39(1):93–107.
15. Hanahan D, Weinberg RA. Hallmarks of cancer: the next generation. Cell 2011; 144(5):646–74.
16. Vermeulen MA, Slaets L, Cardoso F, et al. Pathological characterisation of male breast cancer: results of the EORTC 10085/TBCRC/BIG/NABCG international male breast cancer program. Eur J Cancer 2017;82:219–27.
17. Stefanick ML, Anderson GL, Margolis KL, et al. Effects of conjugated equine estrogens on breast cancer and mammography screening in postmenopausal women with hysterectomy. JAMA 2006;295(14):1647–57.
18. Chia K, O'Brien M, Brown M, et al. Targeting the androgen receptor in breast cancer. Curr Oncol Rep 2015;17(2):4.
19. Wiepjes CM, Nota NM, de Blok CJM, et al. The Amsterdam cohort of gender dysphoria study (1972-2015): trends in prevalence, treatment, and regrets. J Sex Med 2018;15(4):582–90.
20. Asscheman H, Giltay EJ, Megens JA, et al. A long-term follow-up study of mortality in transsexuals receiving treatment with cross-sex hormones. Eur J Endocrinol 2011;164(4):635–42.
21. Asscheman H, Gooren LJG, Eklund PLE. Mortality and morbidity in transsexual patients with cross-gender hormone treatment. Metabolism 1989;9:869–73.
22. van Kesteren PJM, Asscheman H, Megens JAJ, et al. Mortality and morbidity in transsexual subjects treated with cross-sex hormones. Clin Endocrinol 1997;47: 337–42.
23. Dhejne C, Lichtenstein P, Boman M, et al. Long-term follow-up of transsexual persons undergoing sex reassignment surgery: cohort study in Sweden. PLoS One 2011;6(2):e16885.
24. Wierckx K, Elaut E, Declercq E, et al. Prevalence of cardiovascular disease and cancer during cross-sex hormone therapy in a large cohort of trans persons: a case-control study. Eur J Endocrinol 2013;169(4):471–8.
25. Wierckx K, Mueller S, Weyers S, et al. Long-term evaluation of cross-sex hormone treatment in transsexual persons. J Sex Med 2012;9(10):2641–51.
26. Blosnich JR, Brown GR, Wojcio S, et al. Mortality among veterans with transgender-related diagnoses in the Veterans Health Administration, FY2000-2009. LGBT Health 2014;1(4):269–76.
27. Gooren L, Morgentaler A. Prostate cancer incidence in orchidectomised male-to-female transsexual persons treated with oestrogens. Andrologia 2014;46(10): 1156–60.
28. Brown GR, Jones KT. Incidence of breast cancer in a cohort of 5,135 transgender veterans. Breast Cancer Res Treat 2015;149(1):191–8.
29. Brown GR, Jones KT. Mental health and medical health disparities in 5135 transgender veterans receiving healthcare in the Veterans Health Administration: a case-control study. LGBT Health 2016;3(2):122–31.
30. de Blok CJM, Wiepjes CM, Nota NM, et al. Breast cancer in transgender people receiving hormone treatment: results of a nationwide cohort study. Endocr Abstr 2018;56:p955.
31. Deebel NA, Morin JP, Autorino R, et al. Prostate cancer in transgender women: incidence, etiopathogenesis, and management challenges. Urology 2017;110: 166–71.
32. Sharif A, Malhotra NR, Acosta AM, et al. The development of prostate adenocarcinoma in a transgender male to female patient: could estrogen therapy have played a role? Prostate 2017;77(8):824–8.

33. Bonkhoff H. Estrogen receptor signaling in prostate cancer: implications for carcinogenesis and tumor progression. Prostate 2018;78(1):2–10.

34. Wolf-Gould CS, Wolf-Gould CH. A transgender women with testicular cancer: a new twist on an old problem. LGBT Health 2016;3(1):6.

35. Olsen CM, Green AC, Nagle CM, et al. Epithelial ovarian cancer: testing the 'androgens hypothesis'. Endocr Relat Cancer 2008;15(4):1061–8.

36. Grynberg M, Fanchin R, Dubost G, et al. Histology of genital tract and breast tissue after long-term testosterone administration in a female-to-male transsexual population. Reprod Biomed Online 2010;20(4):553–8.

37. Hage JJ, Dekker JJ, Karim RB, et al. Ovarian cancer in female-to-male transsexuals: report of two cases. Gynecol Oncol 2000;76(3):413–5.

38. Dizon DS, Tejada-Berges T, Koelliker S, et al. Ovarian cancer associated with testosterone supplementation in a female-to-male transsexual patient. Gynecol Obstet Invest 2006;62(4):226–8.

39. Taylor ET, Bryson MK. Cancer's margins: trans* and gender nonconforming people's access to knowledge, experiences of cancer health, and decision-making. LGBT Health 2015. https://doi.org/10.1089/lgbt.2015.0096.

40. Stevens EE, Abrahm JL. Adding silver to the rainbow: palliative and end-of-life care for the geriatric LGBTQ patient. J Palliat Med 2018. https://doi.org/10.1089/jpm.2018.0382.

41. Urban RR, Teng NN, Kapp DS. Gynecologic malignancies in female-to-male transgender patients: the need of original gender surveillance. Am J Obstet Gynecol 2011;204(5):e9–12.

42. Schenck TL, Holzbach T, Zantl N, et al. Vaginal carcinoma in a female-to-male transsexual. J Sex Med 2010;7(8):2899–902.

43. Baldassarre M, Giannone FA, Foschini MP, et al. Effects of long-term high dose testosterone administration on vaginal epithelium structure and estrogen receptor-alpha and -beta expression of young women. Int J Impot Res 2013; 25(5):172–7.

44. Baldassarre M, Perrone AM, Giannone FA, et al. Androgen receptor expression in the human vagina under different physiological and treatment conditions. Int J Impot Res 2013;25(1):7–11.

45. Cahill DW, Bashirelahi N, Solomon LW, et al. Estrogen and progesterone receptors in meningiomas. J Neurosurg 1984;60:985–93.

46. Blankenstein MA, Verheijen FM, Jacobs JM, et al. Occurence, regulation, and significance of progesterone receptors in human meningioma. Steroids 2000; 65:795–800.

47. Sarkar DK. Genesis of prolactinomas: studies using estrogen-treated animals. Front Horm Res 2006;35:32–49.

48. Nota NM, Wiepjes CM, de Blok CJM, et al. The occurrence of benign brain tumours in transgender individuals during cross-sex hormone treatment. Brain 2018;141(7):2047–54.

49. Gil M, Oliva B, Timoner J, et al. Risk of meningioma among users of high doses of cyproterone acetate as compared with the general population: evidence from a population-based cohort study. Br J Clin Pharmacol 2011;72(6):965–8.

50. Driak D, Samudovsky M. Cervical cancer in a female-to-male trans-sexual. Eur J Cancer 2004;40(11):1795.

51. Cranston RD, Carballo-Dieguez A, Gundacker H, et al. Prevalence and determinants of anal human papillomavirus infection in men who have sex with men and transgender women. Int J STD AIDS 2018. https://doi.org/10.1177/0956462418797864.

52. Thompson AB, Gillespie SE, Mosunjac MB, et al. Prevalence of anal squamous intraepithelial lesions in HIV-1-infected young men who have sex with men and transwomen. J Low Genit Tract Dis 2018;22(4):340-7.

53. Fein LA, Rosa Cunha I, Slomovitz B, et al. Risk factors for anal dysplasia in transgender women: a retrospective chart review. J Low Genit Tract Dis 2018;22(4): 336-9.

54. Kobayashi T, Sigel K, Gaisa M. Prevalence of anal dysplasia in human immunodeficiency virus-infected transgender women. Sex Transm Dis 2017;44(11): 714-6.

55. Dos Ramos Farias MS, Garcia MN, Reynaga E, et al. First report on sexually transmitted infections among trans (male to female transvestites, transsexuals, or transgender) and male sex workers in Argentina: high HIV, HPV, HBV, and syphilis prevalence. Int J Infect Dis 2011;15(9):e635-40.

56. Loverro G, Di Naro E, Caringella AM, et al. Prevalence of human papillomavirus infection in a clinic sample of transsexuals in Italy. Sex Transm Infect 2016;92(1): 67-9.

57. Hutchison LM, Boscoe FP, Feingold BJ. Cancers disproportionately affecting the New York state transgender population, 1979-2016. Am J Public Health 2018; 108(9):1260-2.

58. Fernandes HM, Manolitsas TP, Jobling TW. Carcinoma of the neovagina after male-to-female reassignment. J Low Genit Tract Dis 2014;18(2):E43-5.

59. Bollo J, Balla A, Rodriguez Luppi C, et al. HPV-related squamous cell carcinoma in a neovagina after male-to-female gender confirmation surgery. Int J STD AIDS 2018;29(3):306-8.

60. tangpricha V, Den Heijer M. Oestrogen and anti-androgen therapy for transgender women. Lancet Diabetes Endocrinol 2017;5(4):291-300.

61. Deutsch MB, Radix A, Wesp L. Breast cancer screening, management, and a review of case study literature in transgender populations. Semin Reprod Med 2017;35(5):434-41.

62. Weyers S, Villeirs G, Vanherreweghe E, et al. Mammography and breast sonography in transsexual women. Eur J Radiol 2010;74(3):508-13.

63. Fenton JJ, Weyrich MS, Durbin S, et al. Prostate-specific antigen-based screening for prostate cancer: evidence report and systematic review for the US preventive services task force. JAMA 2018;319(18):1914-31.

64. US Preventive Task Force, Grossman DC, Curry SJ, Owens DK, et al. Screening for prostate cancer: US preventive services task force recommendation statement. JAMA 2018;319(18):1901-13.

65. Potter J, Peitzmeier SM, Bernstein I, et al. Cervical cancer screening for patients on the female-to-male spectrum: a narrative review and guide for clinicians. J Gen Intern Med 2015;30(12):1857-64.

66. Reisner SL, Deutsch MB, Peitzmeier SM, et al. Test performance and acceptability of self- versus provider-collected swabs for high-risk HPV DNA testing in female-to-male trans masculine patients. PLoS One 2018;13(3):e0190172.

67. Brown B, Poteat T, Marg L, et al. Human papillomavirus-related cancer surveillance, prevention, and screening among transgender men and women: neglected populations at high risk. LGBT Health 2017;4(5):315-9.

68. Newman PA, Roberts KJ, Masongsong E, et al. Anal cancer screening: barriers and facilitators among ethnically diverse gay, bisexual, transgender, and other men who have sex with men. J Gay Lesbian Soc Serv 2008;20(4):328-53.

69. Vogel L. Screening programs overlook transgender people. CMAJ 2014; 186(11):823.

Human Immunodeficiency Virus in Transgender Persons

Cassie G. Ackerley, MD[a,b,*], Tonia Poteat, PhD, MPH, PA-C[c],
Colleen F. Kelley, MD, MPH[a,b,d]

KEYWORDS

- Transgender • Gender identity • Sexual risk behavior • HIV
- Sexually transmitted infections • Preexposure prophylaxis • HIV care continuum
- Hormone therapy

KEY POINTS

- Transgender individuals are vulnerable to stigma, discrimination, and economic marginalization, which can potentiate negative health outcomes, including infection with human immunodeficiency virus (HIV) and other sexually transmitted infections (STIs).
- Regular clinical risk assessments that include a comprehensive sexual history should be used to provide recommendations for HIV and STI screening and to identify individuals who would benefit from HIV preexposure prophylaxis (PrEP).
- PrEP should be considered for all individuals at risk for HIV acquisition, including at-risk transgender people, despite limited data regarding efficacy in this population.
- For transgender individuals living with HIV and using feminizing or masculinizing hormone therapy, there is a potential for drug-drug interactions if they are concurrently receiving ART regimens that include certain protease inhibitors, nonnucleoside reverse transcriptase inhibitors, and/or pharmacokinetic enhancers.
- A multidisciplinary health care approach that integrates individualized, gender-affirming care with HIV prevention and treatment services is essential for addressing the medical and sexual health care needs among transgender individuals.

Disclosure Statement: Dr T. Poteat has received research grants to her institution from Gilead Sciences and ViiV Healthcare. Dr C.F. Kelley has received research grants to her institution from Gilead Sciences. Dr C.G. Ackerley has nothing to disclose.
[a] Division of Infectious Diseases, Department of Medicine, Emory University School of Medicine, Atlanta, GA, USA; [b] The Hope Clinic of the Emory Vaccine Center, 500 Irvin Ct, Suite 200, Decatur, GA 30030, USA; [c] Center for Health Equity Research, University of North Carolina School of Medicine, 333 South Columbia Street, 345B MacNider Hall, Chapel Hill, NC 27514, USA; [d] Department of Epidemiology, Rollins School of Public Health, Emory University, Atlanta, GA, USA
* Corresponding author. The Hope Clinic of the Emory Vaccine Center, 500 Irvin Ct, Suite 200, Decatur, GA 30030.
E-mail address: cmgrims@emory.edu

INTRODUCTION

The burden of human immunodeficiency virus (HIV) disease and other sexually transmitted infections (STIs) among transgender populations is high. Transgender individuals are particularly vulnerable to stigmatization and economic marginalization, which can potentiate negative health outcomes, including HIV.[1,2] The impact of widespread discrimination on psychosocial and economic determinants of health directly influences sexual risk behavior and, in turn, HIV transmission.[2] Despite high rates of HIV infection, particularly among transfeminine individuals, the transgender population remains underserved in terms of medical care and underrepresented in HIV research. In this article, the authors describe the prevalence of HIV infection among transgender groups, present key risk factors associated with HIV acquisition, summarize the data on HIV treatment outcomes, and emphasize the importance of implementing effective HIV prevention and treatment interventions to reduce further HIV transmission and improve morbidity and mortality for transgender people living with HIV disease.[a]

HUMAN IMMUNODEFICIENCY VIRUS INCIDENCE AND PREVALENCE AMONG TRANSGENDER POPULATIONS

HIV prevalence data for transgender populations must be interpreted within the context of widespread stigma and pervasive discrimination. A confluence of structural, social, biological, and individual level factors intersect producing social inequities, including high rates of unemployment, poverty, and homelessness among transgender people that negatively impact health outcomes and perpetuate HIV transmission.[2,4] Reliable estimates of the burden of HIV infection among transgender populations are lacking because gender identity is not uniformly collected in national HIV surveillance reports.[5] Nonetheless, data from meta-analyses, national surveys, multicity, and single-city studies suggest high incidence and prevalence rates of HIV infection in the United States among transgender populations, with the greatest impact among transfeminine individuals.[5] Among more than 3 million HIV testing events reported to Centers for Disease Control and Prevention (CDC) in 2016, the percentage of transgender individuals with a new diagnosis of HIV was more than 3 times the national average.[6] A meta-analysis from 2013 found the HIV seroprevalence of transfeminine adults in the United States to be 22% with a 34-fold increased odds of HIV infection relative to the general population.[7] A more recent systematic review identified 21 studies published between 2012 and 2015 reporting HIV prevalence data for the transfeminine and transmasculine populations.[4] Self-reported HIV prevalence for transfeminine adults ranged from 2% to 29% compared with laboratory-confirmed prevalence of 35% and 40% from 2 studies conducted within large urban settings. As observed in multiple studies,[8] this discrepancy between self-reported and laboratory-confirmed HIV infection in transfeminine populations suggests that there is a substantial proportion of individuals unaware of or unwilling to disclose their HIV status.[2]

Historically, transmasculine individuals have not been considered a group at elevated risk for HIV acquisition because self-reported and laboratory-confirmed

---

[a] In this review, the authors have elected to use the terms "transfeminine" and "transmasculine" in an attempt to be most inclusive of individuals who are on the spectrum of female or male identity, respectively. Alternate terms, such as "transgender women," will be used when describing study populations as defined by these primary data sources.[3]

prevalence has ranged from 0% to 4%.[4,9,10] Notably, a recent analysis of data reported to the National HIV Surveillance System indicated that 15% of transgender people newly diagnosed with HIV from 2009 through 2014 were transmasculine individuals.[11] Despite a growing repository of HIV data on transgender populations, incidence and prevalence estimates must be interpreted with caution because of frequently observed study limitations, such as small sample sizes and use of nonprobability sampling approaches, which increase the likelihood of enrolling participants from high-risk settings.[4]

Importantly, black and Hispanic/Latina transfeminine people in the United States face a disproportionate HIV burden associated with living at the intersection of multiple marginalized identities.[12] A systematic review by Herbst and colleagues[8] reported an HIV seroprevalence rate of 28% among transfeminine adults with an even higher prevalence in black/African American (weighted mean, 56%) compared with white (weighted mean, 17%) or Hispanic/Latina (weighted mean, 16%) individuals. These results were corroborated by a recent analysis of transfeminine people newly diagnosed with HIV infection at CDC-funded sites throughout the United States, where approximately one-half (51%) were black/African American and almost one-third (29%) were Hispanic/Latina.[11] Black and Hispanic/Latina transfeminine people experience discrimination within a context of systemic racism and transphobia that potentiates economic and social inequities, which then contribute to greater vulnerability to HIV infection.[4]

Globally, HIV disparities among transfeminine and transmasculine groups mirror those found in the United States. Based on reports from 15 countries, the pooled HIV prevalence among transfeminine populations was 19%.[7] In recent studies derived from Latin American and southern Asian countries, there were similarly high prevalences of HIV among transfeminine individuals with 14% to 34% prevalence in parts of Latin America and the Caribbean, 18% in India, and an estimated 6% to 22% in Pakistan.[4] The global HIV prevalence among transmasculine populations remains largely unknown because of insufficient investigation. An HIV prevalence of 0% to 2% was reported in a systematic review that included 5 studies performed outside of the United States; however, the validity of these results may have been affected by small sample sizes of less than 100 participants in 4 out of 5 publications and by the use of self-reported HIV status without laboratory confirmation in 3 out of 5 studies.[4] Limited HIV prevalence data from critical areas with ongoing HIV epidemics, including sub-Saharan Africa, central Asia, and Eastern Europe, underscore the urgent need for further inquiry to better understand the burden of HIV disease among transfeminine and transmasculine populations worldwide.[4,7]

SEXUALITY AND HUMAN IMMUNODEFICIENCY VIRUS RISK AMONG TRANSGENDER POPULATIONS

An important component of providing quality health care is ascertaining an individual's sexual orientation, regardless of their gender identity.[13] A diversity of sexual identities have been reported by transfeminine and transmasculine individuals, including heterosexual or opposite-gender, lesbian/gay or same-gender, pansexual, bisexual, queer, and asexual orientations, among others.[14,15] In addition, the types of sex and levels of HIV risk may vary among transgender people.[4,16]

Emerging literature has provided limited data on patterns of sexual behavior among transgender individuals at risk for HIV. Research suggests that most sexually active transfeminine adults and adolescents engage primarily in receptive anal intercourse,[13,17] and condomless receptive anal intercourse with serodiscordant partners confers a high probability of HIV acquisition.[18] Among transfeminine individuals who use feminizing hormones and retain a penis, receptive anal intercourse may be more common than insertive penile intercourse because of difficulty maintaining an erection because of hormonal effects.[13] In addition, receptive anal intercourse may be perceived as more feminine or gender-affirming than insertive intercourse,[13,19] and significant barriers exist in accessing gender-affirming surgeries, such as vaginoplasty.[20] Transmasculine individuals have a range of sexual orientations and sexual practices, including sex with cisgender men and transgender women with penises. These data raise concerns for HIV acquisition risk related to sex with individuals from populations that have a high burden of HIV infection.[9,21–23] In addition, testosterone use by transmasculine individuals can lead to vaginal dryness and atrophy, thus increasing the risk for HIV acquisition during condomless vaginal intercourse.[4,24]

Elevated frequencies of condomless sex, sex with multiple partners, and transactional sex have been reported among transfeminine individuals.[5,8] Based on survey data among transfeminine participants in 3 major US cities, the estimated prevalence of sex work was 44%.[25] Individuals involved in these transactional sex networks are at greater risk for exposure to HIV and other STIs, yet financial hardships that result from discrimination and economic marginalization may leave individuals without other viable employment options.[24,26] Furthermore, the criminalization of sex work in the United States limits negotiation power for condom use and also places individuals at greater risk for rape or sexual assault, thereby increasing the likelihood of exposure to HIV.[17,27,28] Higher rates of incarceration as a consequence of criminalized sex work may further facilitate HIV risk by perpetuating economic difficulties, limiting health care access, and increasing social stigma. An emerging body of literature on sexual behaviors among some transmasculine people describe HIV risk primarily related to condomless receptive anal and vaginal intercourse,[9,21] use of alcohol or other substances during sex, as well as challenges with negotiating safer sex practices due to unequal interpersonal power dynamics.[24,29]

Psychosocial health problems, including depression and suicidality, polysubstance abuse, intimate partner violence, and victimization, are disproportionately experienced by transgender individuals.[30] Impaired reasoning and decreased inhibition related to alcohol and drug use before or during sex may subsequently lead to engagement in higher-risk sexual practices.[26] Approximately 60% of transgender people have been victims of violence or harassment, most commonly as a result of transphobia and/or gender-based discrimination.[14,31] Sexual assault has been experienced by an estimated 21% of transfeminine and transmasculine individuals,[8,31] compared with 19% of cisgender women and 1.5% of cisgender men.[32] Coerced sex, forced sex, and intimate partner violence typically preclude safer sex negotiations, thereby increasing the risk of HIV transmission if the perpetrator is living with HIV.[26] Both polysubstance abuse and intimate partner violence have been found to be associated with sexual risk behavior, thus contributing to HIV vulnerability.[30]

Performing regular clinical risk assessments that screen for violence and include a comprehensive sexual history is integral to providing appropriate medical care for transgender individuals and should be performed in an open and nonjudgmental way that establishes respect for the patient and yields trust in the provider. Following the principles of trauma-informed care,[33] providers should respond to disclosures of recent or past abuses with empathy and support. Based on the circumstances, further specific actions may be warranted, such as safety planning; linkage to safe housing, law enforcement, legal, or community resources; or referrals to individual and/or group counseling.[33] As with all individuals, diversity of sexual identities and practices necessitates the use of a patient-centered approach to recommendations for HIV/STI screening and in determining which individuals will optimally benefit from preexposure prophylaxis (PrEP), discussed further in a later section (Fig. 1).

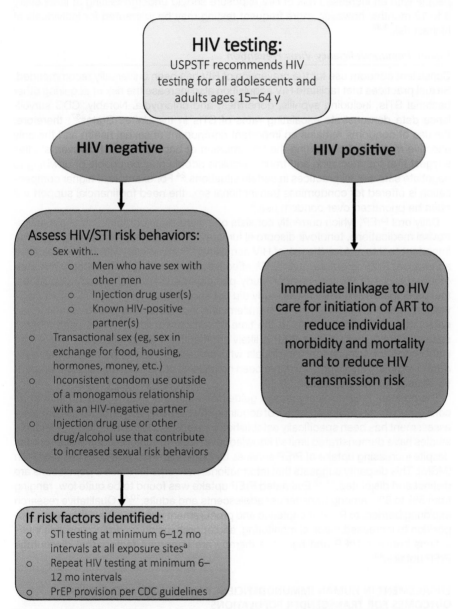

Fig. 1. A suggested algorithm for evaluation of HIV status and HIV/STI risk behavior among transgender people. [a] Oropharyngeal, vaginal, urethral, and/or rectal sites. USPSTF, US Preventive Services Task Force.

HUMAN IMMUNODEFICIENCY VIRUS TESTING AND PREVENTION
Human Immunodeficiency Virus Testing

The US Preventive Services Task Force recommends that all adolescents and adults 15 to 65 years of age be screened at least once for HIV infection regardless of their level of exposure risk.[34] Per CDC national guidelines, individuals at increased risk for HIV should be screened at least annually.[35] In the authors' opinion, transgender people with an increased risk of HIV exposure should undergo testing at least every 6 to 12 months; however, more frequent testing may be warranted for individuals at highest risk.[3,36]

Human Immunodeficiency Virus Prevention

Consistent condom use for the prevention of HIV has been universally recommended. Sexual practices that facilitate HIV acquisition also increase the risk of acquiring other bacterial STIs, including syphilis, gonorrhea, and chlamydia. Notably, CDC surveillance data demonstrate escalating rates of STIs in the United States[37]; therefore, the use of condoms remains an important component of sexual health and the only effective method of preventing the transmission of bacterial STIs. However, studies suggest that transfeminine and transmasculine people may be unable or unwilling to negotiate safe sexual practices in certain situations.[24] For example, if higher compensation is offered for condomless transactional sex, the need for financial support will often be prioritized over condom use.[5]

Daily oral PrEP, which currently consists of a fixed-dose combination of the antiretroviral medications, tenofovir disoproxil fumarate (TDF) and emtricitabine (FTC), is an important tool to reduce the risk of HIV acquisition.[38] In general, with daily medication adherence, PrEP is greater than 90% effective at preventing HIV infection.[39] A subgroup analysis of the transgender study participants (14% of the study population) that participated in the iPrEX Ole study did not show efficacy of TDF-FTC for HIV prevention; however, none of the 11 transfeminine individuals diagnosed with HIV had detectable plasma drug levels at the time of seroconversion.[40] It has been inferred based on these findings that PrEP is likely an effective and beneficial HIV prevention intervention for transgender individuals who can adhere to the recommended daily dosing regimen, although there have been no trials as of yet to demonstrate therapeutic efficacy for this population.[40]

The national PrEP clinical practice guidelines state that PrEP utilization should be considered for all individuals at risk of acquiring HIV sexually, yet no formal risk behavior assessment has been specifically established for transgender individuals.[38,40] Multiple studies have demonstrated limited knowledge about PrEP among transgender groups despite increasing uptake of PrEP services by cisgender men who have sex with men (MSM). This disparity suggests that informational networks for these 2 populations are distinct and disjointed.[41,42] Estimated PrEP uptake was found to be quite low, ranging from 5% to 8%, among transgender adolescents and adults.[10,42] Qualitative research exploring barriers to PrEP acceptance and procurement suggests that HIV stigma, opposition to increased medical monitoring, and apprehension regarding possible interactions between PrEP and hormone therapy are important factors that discourage PrEP uptake.[43]

ENGAGEMENT IN HUMAN IMMUNODEFICIENCY VIRUS CARE AND CLINICAL OUTCOMES FOR TRANSGENDER POPULATIONS

Transgender individuals often face stigma, discrimination, and poverty that may prevent adequate access to necessary health care services.[14] When seeking HIV-related health care services, compounding factors may discourage HIV-positive transgender individuals from engaging in and remaining in care, including fear and shame associated with the diagnosis, concerns about legal repercussions related to the circumstances by which the infection was acquired, and apprehension regarding potential interactions of antiretroviral therapy (ART) with hormone therapy.[44]

With the introduction of combination ART, HIV-associated morbidity and mortality have declined dramatically due to inhibition of viral replication with subsequent immune reconstitution, thus transforming HIV into a treatable chronic disease.[45,46] Life expectancy for people living with HIV who remain adherent to lifelong ART now closely mirrors that of the uninfected US population.[47] Another important aspect of HIV care is the concept of "treatment as prevention" whereby ART is used for preventing HIV transmission by decreasing the infectivity of the HIV-positive sexual partner among serodiscordant couples.[48] Studies to date have demonstrated zero risk of HIV transmission among serodiscordant heterosexual and male couples in which the HIV-positive partner maintained an undetectable HIV viral load on ART.[49,50] These results have important public health implications for HIV prevention, especially for individuals who are part of those sexual networks disproportionately affected by high HIV prevalence.

The HIV care continuum is a model characterizing health outcomes for individuals living with HIV. The stages of the HIV care continuum include linkage to care following diagnosis, initiation of ART, retention in ongoing HIV medical care services, and ultimately, the achievement and maintenance of virologic suppression.[10,51] Early studies evaluating these HIV-related health outcomes for transfeminine adults revealed fewer individuals were being prescribed ART, and those who received ART had lower rates of adherence compared with cisgender adults.[52,53] Findings from a more recent publication demonstrated that similar proportions of HIV-positive transgender individuals were retained in care (80%), receiving ART (76%) and achieving viral suppression (68%) compared with cisgender men and women.[54] Increased patient and health care provider awareness of HIV risk factors, improvements in access to care, and simpler, more tolerable ART regimens may have contributed to these observed changes over time.[54]

Despite a high burden of HIV, there is very little known about the correlates of HIV care continuum outcomes among transfeminine people of color living with HIV disease. In a study by Bukowski and colleagues,[55] where participant surveys and HIV testing were performed for more than 400 black transgender women (BTW), 51% of all HIV-positive participants were unaware of their diagnosis before testing. Of those who were aware of their diagnosis, most were linked to HIV medical care (96%) and reported retention in care (96%). Approximately 90% had received an ART prescription and 69% reported an undetectable viral load. BTW with undiagnosed HIV were more likely than HIV-negative BTW to have been previously incarcerated and to report difficulties accessing health care services.[55] In addition, some transfeminine people may avoid HIV testing due to past negative experiences within the health care system and fear of receiving a stigmatized diagnosis.[56] These studies suggest that although BTW may defer HIV testing or experience challenges accessing these services, many will progress along the HIV care continuum once diagnosed and linked to care. Further research is needed to address the barriers that prevent access to HIV testing and treatment services for this population.

DRUG INTERACTIONS BETWEEN ANTIRETROVIRAL MEDICATIONS AND HORMONE THERAPY

Research suggests gender-affirming care (eg, hormone therapy) is frequently prioritized over other health care needs, including HIV prevention and treatment services, particularly if there is concern about potential interactions between hormone therapy and ART or PrEP.[13,40,57] Health care workers providing care for transgender people living with HIV should be aware of potential drug-drug interactions between hormone therapy and antiretroviral agents. Current recommended ART regimens for initial HIV therapy include a protease inhibitor (PI) or an integrase strand transfer inhibitor in combination with a backbone of 2 nucleoside reverse transcriptase inhibitors. Regimens that include certain PIs, nonnucleoside reverse transcriptase inhibitors, and the pharmacologic booster, cobicistat, may have the potential to decrease the plasma levels of available estradiol and testosterone.[58] Therefore, the use of these antiretroviral agents in conjunction with gender-affirming hormone therapy may require hormone dose adjustments.[58] As with all pharmacologic prescribing, providers are encouraged to check for drug-drug interactions when starting, discontinuing, or switching a medication.

To date, there is no compelling evidence to suggest that TDF-FTC, when used for PrEP or ART, reduces the effectiveness of hormonal contraceptives or feminizing hormone therapy.[59,60] Conversely, studies have not yet fully addressed whether hormonal agents may impact the efficacy of PrEP in preventing HIV transmission. Based on mechanisms of drug metabolism, it has been assumed that TDF and FTC have limited potential for drug-drug interactions such that simultaneous exposure to estrogens and/or progestins would not be expected to interfere with the levels of these drugs.[40] Nevertheless, investigators from the iFACT study reported a 13% decrease in tenofovir plasma concentrations when taken concurrently with feminizing hormone therapy, yet these levels remained above the threshold needed to maintain protection from HIV transmission.[61] In another study, researchers found lower rectal tissue concentrations of TDF-FTC metabolites in transgender women on feminizing hormone therapy compared with postmenopausal cisgender women.[62] Further investigation into PrEP efficacy for transgender populations is warranted, because it remains unclear whether potential decreases in plasma and rectal TDF-FTC concentrations related to feminizing hormone therapy may impact efficacy. Current guidelines recommend that transgender individuals at risk for HIV acquisition be offered PrEP and counseled regarding the importance of strict adherence to optimize effectiveness, especially for patients concurrently receiving gender-affirming hormone therapy.

SUMMARY

The interplay between psychosocial, behavioral, and societal factors that potentiate vulnerability to HIV necessitates the design and implementation of multicomponent HIV prevention and treatment efforts for transgender populations.[2] Ideally, these efforts would include education for transgender adults and adolescents regarding HIV risk factors and safer sex practices, improved access to HIV prevention and treatment services, integration of gender-affirming care, including access to hormone therapy, as well as appropriate referrals as needed to mental health resources, substance abuse treatment programs, and social services. A patient-centered, trauma-informed, multidisciplinary health care approach, involving endocrinologists, primary care providers, HIV specialists, and psychologists, as needed, is likely to be the most effective strategy for meeting the diverse needs of transgender individuals. Future research endeavors should prioritize assessing the efficacy of PrEP for transgender populations, including evaluation of TDF-FTC tissue concentrations necessary for protection at potential sites of HIV acquisition in patients concurrently receiving hormone therapy.[63] Further exploration of potential barriers to PrEP acceptability, accessibility, and uptake in populations highly vulnerable to HIV is greatly needed to help develop and implement effective PrEP prevention programming tailored for the needs of specific transgender communities.[22] Finally, for those living with HIV, further investigation is warranted into effective interventions that address barriers to care and subsequent progression through the stages of the HIV care continuum.

REFERENCES

1. Stieglitz KA. Development, risk, and resilience of transgender youth. J Assoc Nurses AIDS Care 2010;21(3):192–206.
2. Operario D, Nemoto T. HIV in transgender communities- syndemic dynamics and a need for multicomponent interventions. J Acquir Immune Defic Syndr 2010; 55(Suppl 2):S91–3.
3. Guidelines for the primary and gender-affirming care of transgender and gender nonbinary people. p. 1–199. Available at: http://transhealth.ucsf.edu/pdf/Transgender-PGACG-6-17-16.pdf. Accessed June 17, 2016.
4. Poteat T, Scheim A, Xavier J, et al. Global epidemiology of HIV infection and related syndemics affecting transgender people. J Acquir Immune Defic Syndr 2016;72(Suppl 3):S210–9.
5. Garofalo R, Kuhns LM, Reisner SL, et al. Behavioral interventions to prevent HIV transmission and acquisition for transgender women: a critical review. J Acquir Immune Defic Syndr 2016;72(Suppl 3):S220–5.
6. Centers for Disease Control and Prevention. CDC-Funded HIV Testing: United States, Puerto Rico and the U.S. Virgin Islands; 2016. Available at: http://www.cdc.gov/hiv/library/reports/index.html. Accessed September 2018.
7. Baral SD, Poteat T, Strömdahl S, et al. Worldwide burden of HIV in transgender women: a systematic review and meta-analysis. Lancet Infect Dis 2013;13(3): 214–22.
8. Herbst JH, Jacobs ED, Finlayson TJ, et al. Estimating HIV prevalence and risk behaviors of transgender persons in the United States: a systematic review. AIDS Behav 2008;12(1):1–17.
9. McFarland W, Wilson EC, Raymond HF. HIV prevalence, sexual partners, sexual behavior and HIV acquisition risk among trans men, San Francisco, 2014. AIDS Behav 2017;21(12):3346–52.
10. Reisner SL, Jadwin-Cakmak L, White Hughto JM, et al. Characterizing the HIV prevention and care continua in a sample of transgender youth in the U.S. AIDS Behav 2017;21(12):3312–27.
11. Clark H, Babu AS, Wiewel EW, et al. Diagnosed HIV infection in transgender adults and adolescents: results from the national HIV surveillance system, 2009-2014. AIDS Behav 2017;21(9):2774–83.
12. Sevelius JM. Gender affirmation: a framework for conceptualizing risk behavior among transgender women of color. Sex Roles 2012;68(11–12):675–89.
13. Clements-Nolle K, Marx R, Guzman R, et al. HIV prevalence, risk behaviors, health care use, and mental health status of transgender persons - implications for public health intervention. Am J Public Health 2001;91(6):915–21.
14. Grant JM, Mottet LA, Tanis J, et al. Injustice at every turn - a report of the national transgender discrimination survey. Washington, DC: National Center for Transgender Equality and National Gay and Lesbian Task Force; 2011.
15. Kuper LE, Nussbaum R, Mustanski B. Exploring the diversity of gender and sexual orientation identities in an online sample of transgender individuals. J Sex Res 2012;49(2–3):244–54.

16. Operario D, Nemoto T, Iwamoto M, et al. Unprotected sexual behavior and HIV risk in the context of primary partnerships for transgender women. AIDS Behav 2011;15(3):674–82.

17. Nemoto T, Bodeker B, Iwamoto M, et al. Practices of receptive and insertive anal sex among transgender women in relation to partner types, sociocultural factors, and background variables. AIDS Care 2014;26(4):434–40.

18. Baggaley RF, White RG, Boily MC. HIV transmission risk through anal intercourse: systematic review, meta-analysis and implications for HIV prevention. Int J Epidemiol 2010;39(4):1048–63.

19. Melendez RM, Pinto R. 'It's really a hard life': love, gender and HIV risk among male-to-female transgender persons. Cult Health Sex 2007;9(3):233–45.

20. Puckett JA, Cleary P, Rossman K, et al. Barriers to gender-affirming care for transgender and gender nonconforming individuals. Sex Res Social Policy 2018;15(1): 48–59.

21. Kenagy GP, Hsieh CM. The risk less known: female-to-male transgender persons' vulnerability to HIV infection. AIDS Care 2005;17(2):195–207.

22. Mayer KH, Grinsztejn B, El-Sadr WM. Transgender people and HIV prevention-what we know and what we need to know, a call to action. J Acquir Immune Defic Syndr 2016;72(Suppl 3):S207–9.

23. Fisher CB, Fried AL, Desmond M, et al. Facilitators and barriers to participation in PrEP HIV prevention trials involving transgender male and female adolescents and emerging adults. AIDS Educ Prev 2017;29(3):205–17.

24. Neumann MS, Finlayson TJ, Pitts NL, et al. Comprehensive HIV prevention for transgender persons. Am J Public Health 2017;107(2):207–12.

25. Schulden JD, Song B, Barros A, et al. Rapid HIV testing in transgender communities by community-based organizations in three cities. Public Health Rep 2008; 123(Suppl 3):101–14.

26. De Santis JP. HIV infection risk factors among male-to-female transgender persons: a review of the literature. J Assoc Nurses AIDS Care 2009;20(5):362–72.

27. Guadamuz TE, Wimonsate W, Varangrat A, et al. HIV prevalence, risk behavior, hormone use and surgical history among transgender persons in Thailand. AIDS Behav 2011;15(3):650–8.

28. Shannon K. HIV prevention, criminalization, and sex work: where are we at? 2016. Available at: https://www.catie.ca/en/pif/fall-2016/hiv-prevention-criminalization-and-sex-work-where-are-we. Accessed September 28, 2018.

29. Sevelius J. "There's no pamphlet for the kind of sex I have": HIV-related risk factors and protective behaviors among transgender men who have sex with non-transgender men. J Assoc Nurses AIDS Care 2009;20(5):398–410.

30. Brennan J, Kuhns LM, Johnson AK, et al. Syndemic theory and HIV-related risk among young transgender women: the role of multiple, co-occurring health problems and social marginalization. Am J Public Health 2012;102(9): 1751–7.

31. Lombardi EL, Wilchins RA, Priesing D, et al. Gender violence. J Homosex 2002; 42(1):89–101.

32. Smith SG, Chen J, Basile KC, et al. The national intimate partner and sexual violence survey (NISVS): 2010-2012 state report. Atlanta (GA): National Center for Injury Prevention and Control, Centers for Disease Control and Prevention; 2017.

33. Machtinger EL, Cuca YP, Khanna N, et al. From treatment to healing: the promise of trauma-informed primary care. Womens Health Issues 2015;25(3):193–7.

34. Human immunodeficiency virus (HIV) infection: screening. Home - US Preventive Services Task Force; 2013. Available at: www.uspreventiveservicestaskforce.org/Page/Document/UpdateSummaryFinal/human-immunodefieciency-virus-hiv-infection-screening.

35. Branson BM, Handsfield HH, Lampe MA, et al. Revised recommendations for HIV testing of adults, adolescents, and pregnant women in health-care settings. MMWR Recomm Rep 2006;55(RR14):1–17.

36. Bachmann LH. Sexually transmitted infections in HIV-infected adults and special populations: a clinical guide. Cham (Switzerland): Springer; 2017. Available at: https://login.proxy.library.emory.edu/login?url=http://search.ebscohost.com/login.aspx?direct=true&db=nlebk&AN=1534778&site=ehost-live&scope=site. Accessed September 27, 2018.

37. Centers for Disease Control and Prevention. Sexually Transmitted Disease Surveillance 2016. Atlanta: U.S. Department of Health and Human Services; 2017.

38. Centers for Disease Control and Prevention. US public health service: preexposure prophylaxis for the prevention of HIV infection in the United States—2017 update: a clinical practice guideline. Available at: https://www.cdc.gov/hiv/pdf/risk/prep/cdc-hiv-prep-guidelines-2017.pdf. Accessed September 1, 2018.

39. Grant RM, Lama JR, Anderson PL, et al. Preexposure chemoprophylaxis for HIV prevention in men who have sex with men. N Engl J Med 2010;363(27):2587–99.

40. Deutsch MB, Glidden DV, Keatley J, et al. HIV pre-exposure prophylaxis in transgender women- a subgroup analysis of the iPrEx trial. Lancet HIV 2015;2:e512–9.

41. Wilson EC, Jin H, Liu A, et al. Knowledge, indications and willingness to take pre-exposure prophylaxis among transwomen in San Francisco, 2013. PLoS One 2015;10(6):e0128971.

42. Kuhns LM, Reisner SL, Mimiaga MJ, et al. Correlates of PrEP indication in a multi-site cohort of young HIV-uninfected transgender women. AIDS Behav 2016;20(7):1470–7.

43. Sevelius JM, Keatley J, Calma N, et al. 'I am not a man': trans-specific barriers and facilitators to PrEP acceptability among transgender women. Glob Public Health 2016;11(7–8):1060–75.

44. Dowshen N, Lee S, Franklin J, et al. Access to medical and mental health services across the HIV care continuum among young transgender women: a qualitative study. Transgend Health 2017;2(1):81–90.

45. Simon V, Ho DD, Abdool Karim Q. HIV/AIDS epidemiology, pathogenesis, prevention, and treatment. Lancet 2006;368(9534):489–504.

46. Severe P, Juste MAJ, Ambroise A, et al. Early versus standard antiretroviral therapy for HIV-infected adults in Haiti. N Engl J Med 2010;363(3):257–65.

47. Samji H, Cescon A, Hogg RS, et al. Closing the gap: increases in life expectancy among treated HIV-positive individuals in the United States and Canada. PLoS One 2013;8(12):e81355.

48. Cohen MS, Gay C, Kashuba ADM, et al. Narrative review- antiretroviral therapy to prevent the sexual transmission of HIV-1. Ann Intern Med 2007;146(8):591–601.

49. Rodger AJ, Cambiano V, Bruun T, et al. Sexual activity without condoms and risk of HIV transmission in serodifferent couples when the HIV-positive partner is using suppressive antiretroviral therapy. JAMA 2016;316(2):171–81.

50. Cohen MS, Chen YQ, McCauley M, et al. Prevention of HIV-1 infection with early antiretroviral therapy. N Engl J Med 2011;365(6):493–505.

51. Understanding the HIV care continuum. Centers for Disease Control and Prevention - National Center for HIV/AIDS, Viral Hepatitis, STD and TB Prevention;

2018. Available at: https://www.cdc.gov/hiv/pdf/library/factsheets/cdc-hiv-care-continuum.pdf.

52. Melendez RM, Exner TA, Ehrhardt AA, et al. Health and health care among male-to-female transgender persons who are HIV positive. Am J Public Health 2006; 96(6):1034–7.

53. Sevelius JM, Carrico A, Johnson MO. Antiretroviral therapy adherence among transgender women living with HIV. J Assoc Nurses AIDS Care 2010;21(3): 256–64.

54. Yehia BR, Fleishman JA, Moore RD, et al. Retention in care and health outcomes of transgender persons living with HIV. Clin Infect Dis 2013;57(5):774–6.

55. Bukowski LA, Chandler CJ, Creasy SL, et al. Characterizing the HIV care continuum and identifying barriers and facilitators to HIV diagnosis and viral suppression among black transgender women in the United States. J Acquir Immune Defic Syndr 2018;79(4):413–20.

56. Sevelius JM, Patouhas E, Keatley JG, et al. Barriers and facilitators to engagement and retention in care among transgender women living with human immunodeficiency virus. Ann Behav Med 2014;47(1):5–16.

57. Grant RM, Sevelius JM, Guanira JV, et al. Transgender women in clinical trials of pre-exposure prophylaxis. J Acquir Immune Defic Syndr 2016;72(Suppl 3): S226–9.

58. Guidelines for the use of antiretroviral agents in adults and adolescents living with HIV. Department of health and human services. Available at: http://www.aidsinfo.nih.gov/ContentFiles/ AdultandAdolescentGL.pdf. Accessed September 14, 2018.

59. Murnane PM, Heffron R, Ronald A, et al. Pre-exposure prophylaxis for HIV-1 prevention does not diminish the pregnancy prevention effectiveness of hormonal contraception. AIDS 2014;28(12):1825–30.

60. Highleyman L. PrEP does not lower feminising hormone level in transgender woman 2018. Available at: http://www.aidsmap.com/PrEP-does-not-lower-feminising-hormone-level-in-transgender-women/page/3313080/. Accessed September 2, 2018.

61. Hiransuthikul A, Himmad K, Kerr S, et al. Drug-drug interactions between the use of feminizing hormone therapy and pre-exposure prophylaxis among transgender women: the iFACT study. Paper presented at: AIDS2018. Amsterdam, Netherlands, July 23–27, 2018.

62. Cottrell ML, Prince HM, Maffuid K, et al. Altered TDF/FTC pharmacology in a transgender female cohort: implications for PrEP. Paper presented at: AIDS2018. Amsterdam, Netherlands, July 23–27, 2018.

63. Anderson PL, Reirden D, Castillo-Mancilla J. Pharmacologic considerations for preexposure prophylaxis in transgender women. J Acquir Immune Defic Syndr 2016;72(Suppl 3):S230–4.

Education Needs of Providers of Transgender Population

Lin Fraser, EdD[a],*, Gail Knudson, MD, MEd, FRCPC[b]

KEYWORDS

- Transgender • Trans • Medical education • Barriers to care • Endocrinology
- Transition • Competency

KEY POINTS

- A primary barrier to accessing care is a lack of education in this rapidly evolving field.
- A comprehensive, interdisciplinary, evidence-based training program is needed to respond to these educational needs.
- Training should be based on medicine, mental health, and human rights.
- The World Professional Association for Transgender Health has developed a foundational and advanced competency-based clinical training program in transgender health care.
- The 4 competency domains are caregiver/care receiver relationship, content knowledge across the lifespan, interdisciplinary practice, and professional responsibility/ethics.

INTRODUCTION

The field of trans health is fast growing, interdisciplinary, and global,[1] and the education needs of providers are also growing to keep apace of this expanding discipline.[2,3]

BARRIERS TO CARE

Scant education on the topic of trans health is available in medical school curricula,[2–8] so newly minted physicians and other health care professionals are receiving limited training in this burgeoning field. Most practicing physicians are also not equipped to respond to the needs of their trans patients.[2,4,5] Moreover, research indicates that trans people suffer significant health disparities[6,7,9–19] and have apprehensions regarding even seeking medical care owing to stigma[17–23] and lack of access[7,14–16] to providers sufficiently knowledgeable on the topic.[15] Well-meaning and responsible

Disclosure Statement: No financial interests for either author.
[a] Private Practice, 204 Clement Street, San Francisco, CA 94118, USA; [b] Faculty of Medicine, University of British Columbia, #201 1770 Fort Street, Victoria, BC V8R 1J5, Canada
* Corresponding author.
E-mail address: linfraser@gmail.com

Endocrinol Metab Clin N Am 48 (2019) 465–477
https://doi.org/10.1016/j.ecl.2019.02.008
0889-8529/19/© 2019 Elsevier Inc. All rights reserved.

practitioners do not know what they need to know to provide competent and ethical care[3,24] nor do they know how to access training.

Solution to the Problem

To meet the needs of this diverse and marginalized population, providers of trans health need to stay abreast of the broad learning that does exist as well as education specific to their individual disciplines.[2,24] They will need to maintain the knowledge, skills, and awareness[25,26] relative to both the general and of the specific concerns of this population. They will also need to stay informed of the ethical challenges and issues of personal responsibility within the field,[24,27] because experts differ on some aspects of trans health. Hence, any response to these education needs must take all of these aspects (broad, specific, and ethical) into account.[24,27]

Summary of the Article

To put these needs into context and as an overview, this article begins with a brief history of the field, including the background and need for education[1] and a review of the relevant literature. It then summarizes the educational needs of providers, of what providers need to understand. The following section describes ways in which to respond to these needs via comprehensive, competent, and evidenced-based education and training, primarily developed by the World Professional Association for Transgender Health (WPATH), via their Standards of Care (SOC) guidelines[24,28–34] and the domain-based interdisciplinary Global Education Initiative (GEI) training courses.[24,34–37] Although WPATH is the primary organization that meets the educational needs of interdisciplinary providers, the clinical practice guideline by the Endocrine Society entitled "Endocrine Treatment of Gender-Dysphoric/Gender-Incongruent Persons,"[38,39] in partnership with WPATH, provide more specific guidelines for endocrinologists than the more global and interdisciplinary SOC.

Two cases, 1 simple and 1 complex, are described, with the intent of showing how the GEI competencies work together in the treatment of individuals who might come to an endocrinology practice.

The conclusion discusses the next steps to address the gaps in the education needs of providers of the transgender population.

BACKGROUND AND HISTORY OF EDUCATION
Brief History of the Field

The Harry Benjamin International Gender Dysphoria Association and the early Standards of Care

The field of trans health as a medical discipline is relatively young, starting when a small group of pioneering interdisciplinary professionals founded the Harry Benjamin International Gender Dysphoria Association (HBIGDA) at a conference held by this association in San Diego in 1979.[1] These providers also published the first SOC,[28–34,40] guidelines on how to medically treat patients who suffered from and had been diagnosed with gender dysphoria, then known as transsexualism, a condition where an incongruence was experienced between the subjective sense of gender and assigned sex.[40,41]

The SOC were developed based on professional consensus given the paucity of evidence other than extremely pathologizing literature.[1,28–34] Unlike these early HBIGDA members, conventional medicine believed that transsexuals suffered from a severe psychological condition, possibly a delusional disorder, and that the treatment was intensive psychotherapy to match the mind to the body.

The founders of the HBIGDA, based on their work with their patients, believed that matching the body to the mind via the triadic sequence of medical interventions, hormones and genital surgery, and living in the preferred gender role could bring relief to their gender dysphoria. Although psychotherapy was a major part of the treatment and letters of referral from mental health professionals were required for hormones and surgery, transsexuals were not deemed mentally ill among members of HBIGDA.[1,28–34,42]

Early education
In addition to conferring with their professional colleagues, this small group of pioneers received their education from their patients by listening to what their patients needed and by believing them. Providers had to trust their clinical judgment, their like-minded professional colleagues, and their patients.[1] The early treatment was based on what is now known as the "sex change" medical model, and the patients fit into a binary system of gender, they were male or female, a man or a woman. Much has changed over the years in the sense that gender is now seen as a continuum,[39] although the medical treatment has generally remained the same with the goal to align the body with the mind.

Progression of the Field

Versions, name, and growth
There are 7 versions of the SOC, the first being published in 1979 and the most recent in 2012.[29] Version 8 is in progress, with an evidence-based focus, and will mirror the Endocrine Society Guidelines in its scientific rigor, but will have a broader scope. Because there remains a dearth of research knowledge in the field, many of the recommendations are still based on professional consensus.[43]

As the versions have progressed, there has been a movement from treatment (medical interventions to help the person change from one sex to another to the extent possible) to focusing on individualized overall health care.[1,31,33,44] As discussed elsewhere in this article, the concept of a binary gender identity has also moved to one of a spectrum of identities.[45] The concept of one's identity being a disorder as seen in earlier versions of the Diagnostic and Statistical Manual of Mental Disorders and the International Classification of Diseases is no longer recognized. In addition, WPATH has released depathologization statements to this effect.[46] Medical transition is individualized to optimize the overall health care of the individual and is considered medically necessary.[47] Psychotherapy is no longer required and mental health referrals are no longer required for the initiation of hormone therapy.[29]

The name of the organization of the professionals caring for the community also changed from the HBIGDA to the WPATH in 2007.[1] The organization has grown from just a few health care professionals in 1979 to more than 2500 global interdisciplinary professionals in 2019.

The growth in the membership is most likely due to a number of factors, including tiered membership, an increase in the number of and importance of textbooks in transgender health,[1,48] and special issues in prestigious academic journals such as The Lancet,[14,40,49] increased visibility of the field, hosting conferences outside of Western Europe and North America, chaptering (EPATH and USPATH), and expanding educational programs in interdisciplinary clinical care, all grounded by a larger and more efficient organizational structure with a switch to professional management from a university-based model.

Growth in training and education
Education programs in transgender health have usually been restricted to university-based settings. A number of educational programs do exist targeted at providing

introductory knowledge with respect to the transgender community, but do not involve clinical training. WPATH has developed a clinical education training program through the GEI to provide up-to-date knowledge for clinicians and challenge misperceptions among current providers of care.[35] Hosting conferences and training events outside of Western Europe and North America also promotes networking and learning opportunities from a multicultural perspective. Finally, the new WPATH SOC, version 8, now in progress, includes a Chapter on Education, a first in the history of the document, promoting the importance of this area in providing safe, effective care.

REVIEW OF TRANSGENDER HEALTH EDUCATION LITERATURE
Two Areas

Literature on education is limited and exists in primarily 2 areas, namely, describing gaps in education and professional society guidelines.

Gaps in education and barriers to care

The first type of literature describes the gaps in education and barriers to care.[7] These articles agree that the most common problem is access to care owing to a lack of competent providers and recommend education and training as the solution to the problem. These education programs should exist in the undergraduate, postgraduate, and continuing professional development areas. Moreover, transphobia still exists even among providers and many trans people report a history of poor care.[7,11,50] Some refuse to see providers owing to a perception of maltreatment or incompetence and fear of what will happen in health care provider's offices, emergency rooms, and so on.[11] The field is controversial because treatment impacts reproduction, genitalia, the foundation of identity, and some religious beliefs. Some providers are uncomfortable with the appearance of trans bodies and gender expressions. More often than not, these providers do not possess the knowledge, skills, and awareness to provide safe, effective treatment.

Professional guidelines

The second type of literature in education are professional guidelines for care, such as those published by interdisciplinary professional societies such as WPATH SOC[28] (https://www.wpath.org/publications/soc) and/or guidelines geared toward specific disciplines, such as those published by the Endocrine Society[39] (https://www.endocrine.org/topics/transgender-medicine) and the American Psychological Association[51] or guidelines distributed via surgical societies.[52]

The evidence-based Endocrine Society guidelines (https://www.endocrine.org/topics/transgender-medicine) were published in 2017 and all of the authors providing content are senior WPATH members. Most of these authors are also contributing members to the WPATH SOC Version 8. The Endocrine Society offers educational resources for health care providers on their website, including a clinical education module, an educational slide deck, and a guideline pocket card (**Box 1**).

DISCUSSION: CURRENT WORLD PROFESSIONAL ASSOCIATION FOR TRANSGENDER HEALTH WORK

WPATH is responding to the providers needs in education in 2 ways, first, via a new chapter in the SOC on education[44] and second by developing interdisciplinary training courses through the GEI.[35]

Box 1
Recommendations for health care providers

- Take advantage of formal and informal education and training opportunities consistent with the SOC and Endocrine Society Guidelines.
- Participate in networking opportunities with other interdisciplinary providers.
- Keep up to date with the growing literature.
- Listen carefully to and treat their patients with dignity and respect.
- Be aware of their conscious and unconscious biases given the stigma and marginalization of the transgender populations.

Standard of Care 8: Chapter on Education: Recommendations Based on Professional Consensus

As noted, there is scant literature in the field of transgender health education and what literature exists does not extend itself to systematic review. In other words, no studies thus far show a change in health care outcomes based on educational programs. Therefore, the recommendations in this article are consensus based and are made on an advisement ("we advise") level.[43] The following areas are included:

Institutional Climate
All health care workforce members
All health care providers
Voice and communication
Mental health
Medical training
Nursing
Law
Non–health care-specific disciplines and organizations
Global level: United Nations/World Health Organization/World Bank, and others.

Global Education Initiative

The GEI has developed education programming to meet the educational needs of health care providers. The goal of the competency-based training is to enable the clinician to provide comprehensive, competent, evidence-based, and compassionate care (https://www.wpath.org/gei).[35]

History of the global education initiative

Many WPATH members were requesting a formalized transgender health educational program and the need for this was also suggested in 2 background articles to the WPATH SOC Version 7.[42,53] Education was also a direction outlined in the WPATH Strategic Plan from 2013 to 2017, and this direction was incorporated into the current Strategic Plan implemented in 2017.

Starting in 2013, with a vision to meet the defined education need to increase access to care, a small core team composed of WPATH leadership and led by the co-authors and the WPATH management team developed an interdisciplinary training program in trans health that includes foundations and advanced courses based on the SOC. Since the beginning, this core group has met monthly and the co-chairs and staff has met weekly to develop the program. The initial course developers and trainers were co-authors of SOC. The group is now more diverse and includes more trans-identified trainers. The group has met with a specialist consultant as well as with other selected global parties for advice whenever opportunities have arisen. For example, a team of global experts met in Bangkok at the 23rd WPATH symposium in 2014 to define the scope of the program. The group concluded that any comprehensive interdisciplinary education program would need to incorporate medical, mental health, and human rights into the curricula. A second global group of educational experts met at the subsequent symposium in Amsterdam in 2016 and adopted a variation of the domains and competencies from a multicultural education model,[25,54] which the core team then adapted to trans health.

Domains and competencies

The team recommended that to be competent in trans health, a provider would need knowledge, skills and awareness in the following 4 domains:

a. Caregiver/care receiver relationship,
b. Content knowledge across the lifespan,
c. Interdisciplinary practice, and
d. Professional responsibility/ethics.[37]

The GEI Core Team then expanded these into knowledge, skills, and awareness needed for each competency.

Caregiver/care receiver relationship

Knowledge
1. Understand gender identity as 1 component of an individual's entire identity.
2. Recognize evolving language and terminology.

Skills
1. Create a welcoming and safe environment for the development of therapeutic rapport.
2. Identify appropriate communication styles for transgender and gender nonconforming people across cultures.
3. Affirm interpersonal exchanges.

Cultural Awareness
1. Develop a respectful rapport with all individuals.
2. Understand power and balance in caregiver/care receiver relationship.
3. Recognize and respect diversity within the transgender and gender nonconforming culture.

Interdisciplinary practice

Knowledge
1. Recognize the policies within a system or institution of care and how policies impact gender- and trans-related care.
2. Recognize how the policies within your region reimburse clients.
3. Understand specific discipline appropriate trans health care.
4. Understand basics in cross-disciplinary trans health care.
5. Recognize when interdisciplinary care is optimal for a transgender person and how to mitigate circumstances when that service cannot be provided.

Skills
1. Engage and implement the expertise of professionals in various disciplines as related to trans care and transition care.
2. Provide general health care to transgender people.

Cultural Awareness
a. Understand the role transphobia plays in the delivery of care within an institution.

Content knowledge
Knowledge
a. Know basics about the field.
b. Understand general health care for transgender people and across the lifespan.
c. Understand gender health care for nontransitioning people.
d. Understand the evolution of the field.

Skills
a. Incorporate scientific evidence into clinical decision making.
b. Incorporate patient feedback into treatment.

Awareness
a. Recognize power and balance as it relates to client/patient care and decision making.

Professional responsibility
Knowledge
1. Understand confidentiality.
2. Understand the ethical standards for transgender care.
3. Identify gaps in personal knowledge and continue education in the field.
4. Identify current gaps of knowledge in the field.

Skills
1. Negotiate multiple roles of provider including advocacy, teaching, and cultural humility.
2. Identify and implement appropriate communication styles for transgender and gender nonconforming people across cultures.
3. Listen to and affirm experiences of transgender and gender nonconforming people.
4. Create new evidence to promote deeper understanding in the field.

Cultural Awareness
1. Understand the balance of beneficence and nonmaleficence.
2. Advocate for transgender and gender nonconforming people.

These domains and competencies have been used with the permission of WPATH GEI.

Foundations and advanced courses
These 4 competencies form the basis of a 2-day Foundations Course; the subsequent courses are more related to specific content knowledge (advanced mental health, advanced medical, perioperative care, planning and documenting medical transition, voice and communication, and/or professional responsibility/ethics [ethics]).[35] The following video highlights the program in action: https://www.youtube.com/watch?time_continue=7&v=cim2qb4aCl8.[55]

Certification process
WPATH GEI has developed a certification process, a member benefit, that describes the educational needs of interdisciplinary providers in this specialist field. As noted, the main issue is the lack of competent providers to meet the needs of the enlarging trans population. The goal of certification (and the GEI) is to increase access to competent providers who are trained in medical, mental health, and human rights areas and have demonstrated proficiency in the competencies (**Box 2**).

Box 2
To be competent in trans health, a provider needs knowledge, skills and awareness in the following four domains

- Caregiver/care receiver relationship
- Content knowledge across the lifespan
- Interdisciplinary practice and
- Professional responsibility/ethics
- https://www.wpath.org/about-gei

The following is a description of certification that could serve as a model to other training programs, because it takes into account the education needs to be a provider in this population. Although such qualifications as being a WPATH member might not be important to all providers, such requirements as foundational and advanced interdisciplinary courses, spending time in the trans communities, and having supervision or mentorship and even an examination, are the types of educational needs that could be met elsewhere and possibly universally (https://www.wpath.org/gei/certification).[56]

To be eligible for certification, an applicant must:

1. Be a member of WPATH in good standing for 2 years at the time of final examination.
2. Be licensed and board certified (if applicable) in your specialty or the global equivalent.
3. Complete a minimum of 50 hours of credit as indicated:
   - A minimum of 15 continuing education hours in a WPATH Foundations Course.
   - Approximately 10 hours in advanced coursework.
     - Completion of the Mental Health or Medical Advanced Course.
     - Completion of either the Planning and Documenting or Child and Adolescent Workshop.
   - Ten hours of elective coursework outside of WPATH Core Curriculum showing a mapping back to the core competencies.
     - Caregiver–Care Receiver Relationship, Content Knowledge, Interdisciplinary Practice, and Professional Responsibility.
   - Ten hours of mentorship with a WPATH mentor. Mentors will be WPATH-certified members who have gone through the Grandparenting Process (a minimum of 5 years of membership) and have passed the examination. A list of mentorship opportunities will be offered late Spring 2019 in virtual and live formats, and in group or individual settings.
   - Five continuing education hours listening to voices of the transgender, transsexual, and gender nonbinary communities. Examples include attending town halls at GEI conferences, attending designated workshops at WPATH conferences or other approved conferences/workshops, attending local community events, and participating in online education or community forums.
4. Provide evidence of knowledge, skill, and accomplishments in transgender health that is, Curriculum Vitae, publications, case studies, experience, and learning initiatives.
5. Agree to adhere to the WPATH SOC 7 or latest published revision.

6. Agree to comply with the WPATH-approved transgender, transsexual, and gender nonbinary health-related continuing education requirements of 20 hours every 2 years to the maintain certification.
7. Successfully pass the certification examination.

Partnerships

The GEI program is growing globally, having trained more than 2000 providers to date.[36] The GEI is also developing global partnerships with such organizations as the Pan-American Health Organization, UNAIDS International Planned Parenthood Federation, hospitals in the United States such as Mount Sinai and Saint Francis, as well as professional societies of plastic surgery, gynecology, and endocrinology.

Up-to-Date Literature and Educational Opportunities

In addition, up-to-date literature in the field is available in WPATH's journal, the *International Journal of Transgenderism*,[57] biennial symposia, and chapter symposia, as well as the WPATH list serves.

Some other available educational opportunities are as follows. An on-line e-learning pilot project on Transgender Health Education is underway cosponsored by the American Medical Students Association and WPATH GEI led by medical student Masina Wright.[4] University centers as the University of Minnesota offer postgraduate education programs in Transgender Health.[58] Fenway Health offers e-learning modules[59] and the Transgender Echo Program and Callen-Lorde Clinic offer a global internship program. Institutions such as Mount Sinai in New York and Saint Francis in San Francisco are implementing transgender health education by training every member of their institutions in the basics of transgender health care and cultural competency.[60,61] The US Veterans Administration has piloted series of e-consultations with physicians across the United States.[62] The Pan-American Health Organization, in concert with WPATH GEI, is developing an e-learning transgender health course for their online university.[63]

CASES

The following 2 cases, one straightforward and the other more complex, show how the WPATH competencies can work together in the treatment of individuals who might come to the endocrinologist's practice.

Case A

Twenty-five-year-old Ryan identifies as a trans male (assigned female at birth) and socially transitioned 5 years ago. He presents to you requesting masculinizing hormone therapy with a detailed referral from his family physician indicating how he meets the criteria for hormone therapy according to the WPATH SOC 7 criteria as well as the Endocrine Society guidelines. Ryan is healthy and does not have any significant mental or medical health history. He drinks alcohol twice per week and denies any other substance use. He works as a bank teller and lives with his partner of 3 years, Sam, in an apartment in the suburbs.

This case is relatively straightforward. The endocrinologist must first be comfortable providing care to trans patients (care receiver relationship, professional responsibility) and must possess the knowledge (content knowledge) to perform the basic screening tests before the initiation of hormones. The provider must know the appropriate dosages for initiation, iteration, and maintenance of hormones, as well as providing psychoeducation before the initiation of hormones and obtaining informed consent.

The endocrinologist may also engage the family physician (interdisciplinary care) to provide maintenance dosing of testosterone.

Case B

Eighteen-year-old Jan identifies as nonbinary (assigned male at birth) and uses they/them pronouns. Jan is interested in taking feminizing hormones to look more androgynous. They do not want breast growth, but want to feminize their features. They identify as asexual and are not interested in sexual function or sperm preservation. They have been diagnosed with an eating disorder (anorexia) and were hospitalized at age 16 because they were medically unstable. They continue to struggle with this condition, but have maintained their goal weight.

As in the first case, the endocrinologist must examine their comfort level in working with trans patients (professional responsibility, relationship) who present with less conventional features and requests. This case calls on the endocrinologist to have up-to-date knowledge of the various combinations of hormone therapy (content knowledge) to suit the patient's request. They also must be aware that this request is medically possible. The individual may need to be further assessed with respect to their eating disorder in terms of both medical stability and how this intertwines, if indeed so, with their gender identity. The endocrinologist would be wise to consult with the care providers, be they mental health, internal medicine, or adolescent medicine in an interdisciplinary manner to move forward as a team in a safe, effective, and ethical manner (interdisciplinary care).

SUMMARY

Formalized education programs in transgender health care are just beginning. Much more work is left to do, and the field is still on the ground floor when it comes to education. For example, although feedback is quite positive regarding the GEI programs, formal evidence-based outcome studies on the efficacy of the programs need to be conducted. Current plans for GEI include continued global expansion especially in the developing world and building online curricula to increase access. The vision includes developing GEI across continents and countries and continuing partnerships with other institutional curricula, nongovernmental organizations, and ministries of health.

REFERENCES

1. Fraser L. Gender dysphoria: definition and evolution through the years. In: Trombetta C, Liguori G, Bertolotto M, editors. Management of gender dysphoria, a multidisciplinary approach. Milan (Italy): Springer; 2015. p. 19–33.
2. Dubin SN, Nolan IT, Streed CG Jr, et al. Transgender health care: improving medical students' and residents' training and awareness. Adv Med Educ Pract 2018; 9:377–91.
3. Davidge-Pitts C, Nippoldt TB, Danoff A, et al. Transgender health in endocrinology: current status of endocrinology fellowship programs and practicing clinicians. J Clin Endocrinol Metab 2017;102(4):1286–90.
4. Wright M. Trans health leadership course. AMSA; 2018. Available at: https://www.amsa.org/members/career/scholars-programs/trans-health/. Accessed March 17, 2019.
5. Safer JD, Tangpricha V. Out of the shadows: it is time to mainstream treatment for transgender patients. Endocr Pract 2008;14(2):248–50.

6. Lombardi E. Public health and trans people: barriers to care and strategies to improve treatment. In: Meyer E, Northridge ME, editors. The health of sexual minorities public health. New York: Springer; 2007. p. 15.
7. Korpaisarn S, Safer JD. Gaps in transgender medical education among healthcare providers: a major barrier to care for transgender persons. Rev Endocr Metab Disord 2018;19(3):271–5.
8. Breussow D, Poteat T. Primary care providers' role in transgender healthcare. JAAPA 2018;31(2):8–11.
9. Lombardi E. Enhancing transgender health care. Am J Public Health 2001;91(6): 869–72.
10. Bauer GR, Hammond R, Travers R, et al. I don't think this is theoretical: this is our lives: how erasure impacts health care for transgender people. J Assoc Nurses AIDS Care 2009;20:348–61.
11. Grant J, Mottet L, Tanis J, et al. Injustice at every turn: a report of the national transgender discrimination survey. Washington, DC: National Center for Transgender Equality and National Gay and Lesbian Task Force; 2011.
12. Bradford J, Reisner SL, Honnold JA, et al. Experiences of transgender-related discrimination and implications for health: results from the Virginia transgender health initiative study. Am J Public Health 2013;103:1820–9.
13. Giffort D, Underman K. The relationship between medical education and trans health disparities: a call to research. Sociol Compass 2016;10(11):999–1013.
14. Reisner S, Poteat T, Keatley J, et al. Global health burden and needs of transgender populations: a review. Lancet 2016;388(10042):412–36.
15. Safer J, Coleman E, Feldman J, et al. Barriers to health care for transgender individuals. Curr Opin Endocrinol Diabetes Obes 2016;23(2):168–71.
16. Coutin A, Wright S, Li C, et al. Missed opportunities: are residents prepared to care for transgender patients? A study of family medicine, psychiatry, endocrinology and urology residents. Can Med Educ J 2018;9(3):e41–55.
17. Kcomt L. Profound health-care discrimination experienced by transgender people: rapid systematic review. Soc Work Health Care 2019. https://doi.org/10.1080/00981389.2018.1532941.
18. Feldman J, Brown G, Deutsch M, et al. Priorities for transgender medical and healthcare research. Curr Opin Endocrinol Diabetes Obes 2016;23(2):180–7.
19. Valentine S, Shepherd J. A systematic review of social stress and mental health among transgender and gender non-conforming people in the United States. Clin Psychol Rev 2018;66. https://doi.org/10.1016/j.cpr.2018.03.003.
20. Rood B, Reisner S, Surace FI, et al. Expecting rejection: understanding the minority stress experience of transgender and gender nonconforming individuals. Transgend Health 2016;1(1):151–64.
21. Hendricks ML, Testa RJ. A conceptual framework for clinical work with transgender and gender nonconforming clients: an adaptation of the minority stress model. Prof Psychol Res Pr 2012;43(5):460–7.
22. Bockting W, Miner M, Swinburne R, et al. Stigma, mental health and resilience in an online sample of the US transgender population. Am J Public Health 2013; 103(5):943–51.
23. Aravasirikul S, Wilson E. Spilling the T on Trans-misogyny and microaggressions: an intersectional oppression and social process among trans women. J Homosex 2018. https://doi.org/10.1080/00918369.2018.1542203.
24. Fraser L. Integrative and ethical mental health care of transgender and gender non conforming adults. In: Carlozzi A, Choate K, editors. Transgender and

gender diverse persons: a handbook for service providers, educators, and families. New York: Routledge; 2019. p. 93–115.

25. Sue DW, Arredondo P, McDavis RJ. Multicultural counseling competencies and standards: a call to the profession. J Couns Dev 1992;70:477–86.

26. Competencies for counseling with transgender clients. Approved by ALGBTIC Board - September 18, 2009. Approved by American Counseling Association Governing Council- Nov 7, 2009.

27. Beauchamp T, Childress J. Principles of biomedical ethics. 6th edition. New York: Oxford University Press; 2009. p. 12.

28. WPATH website, Standards of Care 7. Available at: https://www.wpath.org/publications/soc. Accessed March 17, 2019.

29. Coleman E, Bockting W, Botzer M, et al. Standards of Care for the health of transsexual, transgender, and gender-nonconforming people, version 7. Int J Transgend 2012;13(4):165–232.

30. Fraser L. Standards of care, transgender health. In: Whelehan P, Bolin A, editors. The international encyclopedia of human sexuality. 1st edition. John Wiley & Sons, LTD Online Library; 2015. p. 496. ISBN-13: 978-1405190060.

31. Coleman E. An overview of the standards of care for the health of transsexual, transgender and gender nonconforming people. In: Ettner R, Monstrey S, Coleman E, editors. Principles of transgender medicine and surgery. 2nd edition. New York: Routledge; 2016. p. 36–42.

32. Fraser L, Knudson G. Past and future challenges associated with standards of care for gender transitioning clients. In: Carroll L, Mizock L, editors. Clinical issues and affirmative treatment with transgender clients, psychiatric clinics of North America. Philadelphia: Elsevier; 2017. p. 15–27.

33. Fraser L, Knudson G. The WPATH Standards of Care. In: Bouman W, Arcelus J, editors. The transgender handbook, a guide for transgender people, their families and professionals. New York: Nova Science Publishers; 2017. p. 201–15.

34. Karasic D, Fraser L. Multidisciplinary care and the standards of care for transgender and gender nonconforming individuals. Clin Plast Surg 2018;45(3):295–9.

35. WPATH. Global Education Initiative. WPATH; 2018. Available at: https://www.wpath.org/gei. Accessed March 17, 2019.

36. History of GEI. Available at: https://www.wpath.org/about-gei. Accessed March 17, 2019.

37. Global Education Initiative. A vision of core competencies for caregivers serving transgender and gender nonconforming people. A pamphlet describing the WPATH GEI core competencies. Chicago: World Professional Association for Transgender Health; 2017. Available at: https://www.wpath.org/about-gei. Accessed March 17, 2019.

38. Hembree WC, Cohen-Kettenis P, Delemarre-van de Waal HA, et al. Endocrine treatment of transsexual persons: an Endocrine Society clinical practice guideline. J Clin Endocrinol Metab 2009;94(9):3132–54.

39. Hembree W, Cohen-Kettenis P, Gooren L, et al. Endocrine treatment of gender dysphoric/gender incongruent persons: an Endocrine Society clinical practice guidelines. J Clin Endocrinol Metab 2017;102(11):1–35.

40. Wylie K, Knudson G, Khan S, et al. Serving transgender people: clinical care considerations and service delivery models in transgender health. Lancet 2016; 388(10042):401–11.

41. Fisk NM. Editorial: gender dysphoria syndrome–the conceptualization that liberalizes indications for total gender reorientation and implies a broadly based multi-dimensional rehabilitative regimen. West J Med 1974;120(5):386–91.

42. Fraser L. Psychotherapy in the world professional association for transgender health's standards of care: background and recommendations. Int J Transgend 2009;11(2):110–27.
43. Knudson, G and Fraser L. SOC 8 Update on Education & Ethics Chapter, WPATH 25th International Symposium, November 6, 2018, Buenos Aires, Argentina.
44. Fraser L, Knudson G. Gender dysphoria and transgender health. In: Wylie K, editor. ABC of sexual health. 3rd edition. Oxford (England): Wiley- Blackwell; 2015. p. 108–11. Available at: https://www.wpath.org/about/history/international-symposia. Accessed March 17, 2019.
45. Bockting W. Psychotherapy and the real life experience: from gender dichotomy to gender diversity. Sexologies 2008;17(4):211–24.
46. WPATH De-psychpathologisation statement. Available at: https://www.wpath.org/policies. Accessed March 17, 2019.
47. Available at: https://www.wpath.org/newsroom/medical-necessity-statement. Accessed March 17, 2019.
48. Ettner R, Monstrey S, Coleman E. Principles of transgender medicine and surgery. 2nd edition. New York: Routledge; 2016.
49. Winter S, Diamond M, Green J, et al. Transgender people: health at the margins of society. Lancet 2016;388(10042):390–400.
50. Poteat T, Park C, Solares D. Changing hearts and minds: results from a multi-country gender and sexual diversity training. PLoS One 2017;12(9):e0184484.
51. American Psychological Association. Guidelines for psychological practice with transgender and gender nonconforming people. Am Psychol 2015;70(9):832–64.
52. Schechter LS, D'Arpa S, Cohen MN, et al. Gender confirmation surgery: guiding principles. J Sex Med 2017;14(6):852–6.
53. Lev AI. The ten tasks of the mental health provider: recommendations for revision of the World Professional Association for Transgender Health's Standards of Care. Int J Transgend 2009;11(2):74–99.
54. ACA 2010 American Counseling Association competencies for counseling with transgender clients. J LGBT Issues Couns 2010;4(3):135–59.
55. Video by Patrick Kelly, used by permission. Available at: https://www.youtube.com/watch?time_continue=6&v=cim2qb4aCl8. Accessed March 17, 2019.
56. Certification process. Available at: https://www.wpath.org/gei/certification. Accessed March 17, 2019.
57. IJT Available at: https://en.wikipedia.org/wiki/International_Journal_of_Transgenderism. Accessed March 17, 2019.
58. University of Minnesota. Available at: https://www.sexualhealth.umn.edu/national-center-gender-spectrum-health. Accessed March 17, 2019.
59. Fenway Health. Available at: https://fenwayhealth.org/the-fenway-institute/. Accessed March 17, 2019.
60. Mount Sinai. Available at: https://www.mountsinai.org/locations/center-transgender-medicine-surgery. Accessed March 17, 2019.
61. Saint Francis. Available at: https://www.dignityhealth.org/bayarea/locations/saintfrancis/services/gender-institute. Accessed March 17, 2019.
62. Kauth MR, Shipherd JC, Lindsay JA, et al. Teleconsultation and training of VHA providers on transgender care: implementation of a multisite hub system. Telemed J E Health 2015;21(12):1012–8.
63. PAHO. Available at: https://www.campusvirtualsp.org. Accessed March 17, 2019.

Moving?

Make sure your subscription moves with you!

To notify us of your new address, find your **Clinics Account Number** (located on your mailing label above your name), and contact customer service at:

Email: journalscustomerservice-usa@elsevier.com

800-654-2452 (subscribers in the U.S. & Canada)
314-447-8871 (subscribers outside of the U.S. & Canada)

Fax number: 314-447-8029

Elsevier Health Sciences Division
Subscription Customer Service
3251 Riverport Lane
Maryland Heights, MO 63043

*To ensure uninterrupted delivery of your subscription,
please notify us at least 4 weeks in advance of move.